Radiology of the Spine

Editor
A. Wackenheim, Strasbourg

B. Wimmer E. Hofmann A. Jacob

Trauma of the Spine

CT and MRI

Foreword by W. Wenz

With 72 Figures in 132 Separate Illustrations

Springer-Verlag Berlin Heidelberg New York
London Paris Tokyo Hong Kong

PD Dr. BERTHOLD WIMMER
Radiologische Klinik
Universität Freiburg
Hugstetter Str. 55
7800 Freiburg i. Br., FRG

Dr. ERICH HOFMANN
Abteilung für Neuroradiologie
in der Kopfklinik
Universität Würzburg
Josef-Schneider-Str. 11
8700 Würzburg, FRG

Dr. AUGUSTINUS L.H. JACOB
Radiologische Klinik
Stadtkrankenhaus
Sauerbruchstr. 7
3180 Wolfsburg, FRG

ISBN-13: 978-3-642-45668-8 e-ISBN-13: 978-3-642-45666-4
DOI: 10.1007/978-3-642-45666-4

Library of Congress Cataloging-in-Publication Data. Wimmer, B. (Berthold), 1938–. Trauma of the spine : computed tomography and nuclear magnetic resonance imaging / B. Wimmer, E. Hofmann, A. Jacob. p. cm. – (Radiology of the spine). Includes bibliographical references.
ISBN 978-3-642-45668-8
1. Spine – Wounds and injuries – Diagnosis. 2. Spine – Tomography. 3. Spine – Magnetic resonance imaging. I. Hofmann, E. (Erich), 1953–. II. Jacob, A. (Augustinus), 1957–. III. Title. IV. Series.
[DNLM: 1. Myelography. 2. Nuclear Magnetic Resonance – diagnostic use. 3. Spinal Cord Injuries – diagnosis. 4. Spinal Injuries – diagnosis. 5. Tomography, X-Ray Computed. WE 725 W757t] RD533.W56 1990
617.3'75044–dc20
DNLM/DLC 89-21887 CIP

Softcover reprint of the hardcover 1st edition 1990

Printed on acid-free paper

Foreword

There is hardly any region of the body where modern imaging techniques have changed the diagnostics of bone lesions as significantly as in the spinal column. Diagnostic innovations have been followed by considerable therapeutic advances.

The authors discuss recent progress in diagnosis using CT and MRI as well as conventional radiological techniques, basing this on their wide experience with patients at the University of Freiburg Hospital, on new biomechanical findings and on the idea that the stability or instability of a vertebral fracture is an essential consideration for successful treatment. They elaborate on their results by providing numerous informative illustrations and statistical studies. They conclude their description by recommending the preferred diagnostic imaging procedures for specific conditions, including the relatively rare indications for myelography.

The determination of the type and sequence of examination is not the only important issue; equally important is to be able to apply it without reflection, specifically in emergency and life-threatening situations. The book has been written by practicing clinicians who are experts prepared to do such examinations at any time for other practicing clinicians. It will be an important aid to all those involved in the diagnosis or therapy of spinal trauma, first of all radiologists, traumatologists, surgeons, and orthopedic surgeons. I wish to recommend that the book be read widely.

W. WENZ

Acknowledgments

The decision to write the present book was made in a day, whereas the idea grew over many months. Working, as we are, in a large institute of radiodiagnostics, it is quite clear that many people will have contributed to the project from behind the scenes.

First of all we want to thank Professor W. Wenz. He supported the plan from the very beginning and helped us in every way - scientifically, technically and organizationally - by allowing us to take advantage of all the possibilities offered by the institute.

It was ideal to be able to publish the book in the series "Radiology of the Spine" founded by Professor A. Wackenheim and we are very grateful for this opportunity.

Our departmental colleagues relieved us of routine duties whenever possible so that we gained many precious hours for work on this book.

The photographer, Mr. Anders, and his team diligently and patiently spent countless hours preparing the illustrations.

We are especially indebted to Mr. B. Lewerich, Dr. J. Wieczorek and other members of the publisher's staff who picked up on the idea at once and, with all their skills, helped make this book a success.

This book is dedicated to our wives and children, who had to do without us quite a few evenings and weekends. Productive work would not have been possible without their love, patience, and approval.

THE AUTHORS

Contents

Introduction

In his conclusion at the end of his excellent book, "Trauma: Conventional Radiographic Study in Spinal Injury", JEAN-CLAUDE DOSCH says: "CT investigations certainly provide additional data by displaying the bone lesions in more detail, thanks to the third dimension ... For our part, we believe that the differentiating power of CT is still insufficient insofar as the structures of the central nervous system are concerned. Perhaps MRI will solve the problem" [23]. In the present book we have attempted to provide an introduction to the analysis of the bony details in CT and to review existing knowledge of the role of MRI in the interpretation of neurologic symptoms.

Any analysis needs criteria. As computed tomography is a radiologic method, we have no other criteria available than those of the conventional image; and what is correct for the one technique cannot be essentially incorrect for the other. We have therefore always preceded the CT findings with the conventional radiographs, even though this may be repetitive for many readers, for the plain film or tomography is the basis of computed tomography and magnetic resonance imaging, and is indispensable for the indications and assessment for the supplementary findings of these techniques. Moreover, this sequence corresponds to the clinical course and so to radiologic development. Recent years have seen a notable expansion in our knowledge of the biomechanics of the vertebral column through clinical and experimental studies, and these have undoubtedly benefited the interpretation of the radiographic findings. This development forms part and parcel of the manifold endeavors towards a reconstructive spinal surgery, based on the principle that the pathologic deformation allows conclusions as to the responsible force, the residual load capacity and the best possible treatment. This addresses the question of fracture stability, and it seems most practicable to base this on the three-column theory of the thoracolumbar spine even though this is not the solution to every problem. Nor is it transferable to the cervical spine, at least not to the atlas and axis.

Our studies have shown that a bony lesion can also be localized by means of signal alteration in MRI, though the detail is significantly better in CT. Therefore, the MRI findings have been included in the relevant chapters only insofar as they provide useful guides.

At the end of the day, the evaluation of CT and MRI in the diagnostics of spinal injury is subject to the fundamental criticism of all imaging techniques: every image reflects only the current state and not the dynamic process in the millisecond of injury. That is why this book is an attempt at analysis and not a dogma. Further investigations and critical considerations are necessary. As WHITE and PANJABI [115] state in their *Guidelines for Biomechanical Interpretation of Radiographs:* "... the oversimplification involved in the use of a static two-dimensional representation of a complicated series of dynamic, three-dimensional events should be kept in mind".

Chapter 1 Basic Considerations

A. Epidemiology and Statistics

Injuries of the spinal column can give rise to severe psychologic, social and economic problems for the injured.

A study of the causes of accidents shows that accidents at work predominate at 33%. 21% result from accidents in the home, another 21% from traffic accidents, and 8% of spinal fractures occur in sport and leisure activities. The remaining 17% occur during various other situations, including the injuries of suicidal attempts [107]. The most comprehensive figures are provided by the statistics of the German official bodies dealing with accidents in terms of occupation: an average of 2942 injuries of the spine are recorded annually. The average period of hospital treatment is 44 days for each patient who is registered as disabled at 135 days [18].

Our own series of cases, which relates to a 5-year period (1981-1985), represents the incidence in a Trauma Unit with a catchment area of some 450000 inhabitants. The analysis of the records of 572 patients shows an anatomic distribution pattern of spinal fractures which is very consistent with other large series (Table 1).

Table 1. Distribution pattern of 814 spinal fractures in 572 patients

	Single segment	Multiple segments	
Cervical	55	2 Segments	26
		3 Segments	5
Thoracic	123	2 Segments	28
		3 Segments	6
		4 Segments	1
Lumbar	220	2 Segments	39
		3 Segments	20
		4 Segments	7
Cervical plus thoracic		2 Segments	5
		3 Segments	1
		7 Segments	1
Cervival plus thoracic and lumbar		4 Segments	1
Thoracic plus lumbar		2 Segments	26
		3 Segments	5
		4 Segments	2
		6 Segments	1
Single segment	398	Multiple segments	174

This shows the familiar typical maximum distribution at the cervicothoracic and thoracolumbar transition zones. Multiple fractures were seen in almost a third of the patients (30.4%). The fact that 42 of these (altogether 7.3% of all patients) had sustained fractures in different parts of the spine proves the need for radiography of all segments. This was also stressed in the review of CALENOFF et al. [12]: a second fracture that has been initially overlooked is only diagnosed after 53 days on average.

A second personal study covering the same period clarifies the role of CT; it was most frequently employed to exclude or demonstrate fractures in the upper and lower cervical region, where conventional radiographs are often accompanied by serious diagnostic difficulties because of superimposition of the skull-base or shoulder-girdle. MEULI finds it "altogether classic" that fractures of the 6th or 7th cervical vertebra should be missed [74] (see Fig. 34).

In the thoracolumbar section, CT has the specific task of assessing the stability of the demonstrated fractures. Because of the lesser diagnostic problems in the conventional images it is less often indicated.

The detail resolution of the CT image is superior to that of the plain film. This leads to greater security in both the demonstration and exclusion

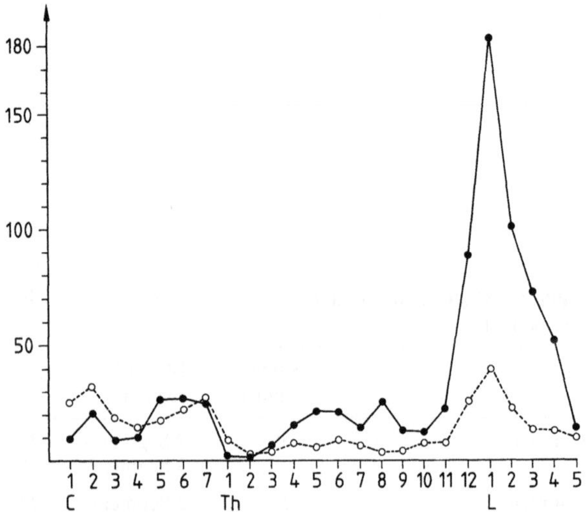

Fig. 1. Survey of investigations of spinal fractures over 5 years. *Continuous line:* conventional radiography only. *Interrupted line:* additional CT imaging of the different segments

of fractures, particularly in the region of the pedicles, articular processes and posterior arch. The findings in a retrospective study of 366 motion segments are listed in Table 2.

The outcome of the improved assessment of the bony injuries is also reflected in the analysis of stability, as shown in Table 3.

Table 2. Evaluation of 366 motion segments on plain films and computed tomography

Findings	Plain film *n*	CT *n*
Fracture	206	227
No fracture	95	131
Uncertain	54	0
Image inadequate	11	8
Total	366	366

Table 3. Coincidence and discrepancy of judgment of stability following plain films and computed tomography

	Computed tomography		
Plain film	Stable	Unstable	Uncertain
Stable	<u>116</u>	19	9
Unstable	1	<u>55</u>	–
Uncertain	4	14	<u>6</u>

Coincident results are underlined

In the majority of cases the spinal injury is not the only result of the injury. Jodoin et al. [50] found that 76% of their patients had other lesions requiring treatment:

Locomotor system	48 %
Craniocerebral injury	22.5%
Abdominal injury	15.5%
Facial skeleton	14 %

(Combinations of the various injuries occurred in some cases).

The incidence of neurologic lesions is given as from 10 to 23% [5]. In our own series there was a neurologic deficit in 13%, and in 44% of those in whom CT was undertaken. There is no close connexion between a narrowing of the spinal canal and a neurologic lesion. This emphasizes the importance of skilled neurologic investigation, and it also indicates the importance of MRI.

B. Descriptive and Sectional Anatomy

The clinical usefulness of computed tomography is based on specially oriented thin axial slices. Ideally, these slices are parallel to the vertebral body end-plate. Magnetic resonance imaging (MRI) allows sections in any spatial orientation.

I. Bones

At birth the vertebra is not yet mature. Apart from the median ossification center of the vertebral body, there exist two lateral centers in the pedicles. The dorsal parts of the arch are completely open. Fusion of the lateral ossification centers is completed only between the ages of 4 and 8 years. The fusion process commences at the lower thoracic spine, spreading in a cranial and caudal direction. The age-dependent developmental status and possible congenital malformations should always be taken into consideration when assessing fractures, especially in the region of the vertebral arches.

With the exception of the first two cervical vertebrae (atlas and axis) a typical vertebra consists of:

- an anterior portion, the vertebral body, and
- a posterior portion, the neural arch, which in turn is divided into:
  - an anteriorly situated pair of pedicles,
  - a pair of superior and a pair of inferior articular processes,
  - a pair of posterolateral laminae,
  - a pair of transverse processes and
  - a single spinous process.

The posterior aspect of the vertebral body and the neural arch together with the pedicles encompass the vertebral foramen. The vertebral foramina form the spinal canal which contains the spinal cord and its surrounding structures. A superior and inferior incisura at the pedicles of successive vertebrae form the intervertebral foramen or canal that harbours the spinal nerve.

The basivertebral vein penetrates the posterior surface of each vertebral body producing a tiny interruption of the cortical surface with a concomitant compaction of bone. In the trabeculation of the spongiosa of the vertebral body, the channels of the basivertebral veins can be clearly distinguished due to their typical arrangement and Y-shape. This allows easy differentiation from fracture [43].

The cervical vertebrae are the smallest of the true vertebrae. The transverse processes of the cervical spine develop from a vertebral and a costal rudiment which after incomplete fusion are still separated by the foramen of the transverse process. These foramina serve as openings for the vertebral artery with its accompanying venous plexuses and for sympathetic nerve structures. The transverse process presents an anterior and posterior tubercle with an interposed sulcus for the spinal nerve. The fifth and sixth cervical vertebrae sometimes exhibit an especially prominent anterior tubercle which must not be confused with spondylosis or a traumatic avulsion in the lateral radiogram. The cervical spinal canal appears approximately triangular in the axial CT scan with the tip of the triangle pointing in a posterior direction. The vertebral bodies of C3-7 are oval and larger in transverse than anteroposterior diameter [43]. The concave superior endplates terminate in lateral protuberances, the uncinate processes, projecting superiorly to the vertebral bodies. These processes form part of the anterior margin of the neural foramen.

The cervical pedicles are short in the axial scan. In the likewise short transverse processes, the transverse foramina can be distinguished.

The atlas, the first cervical vertebra, differs from the other cervical vertebrae by lacking a vertebral body and spinous process and by being ring-shaped. The two anterolaterally located lateral masses are connected by a longer posterior and a shorter anterior arch with their anterior and posterior tubercles respectively. Small midline clefts in the posterior or anterior arch are a normal variant which must not be confused with fracture [54, 57]. The usual position of the vertebral body is occupied by the odontoid process of the next lower vertebra, the axis. The posterior arch has a lateral groove at its upper surface in which travel the atlantal loop of the vertebral artery and the first cervical spinal nerve. This groove may be converted into a "foramen arcuatum" by a bridge of bone. The lateral masses have joint facets that articulate with the occipital condyles superiorly and the axis inferiorly.

The central part of the atlas fuses with the body of the axis to form the odontoid process. The intervertebral disk at C1-C2 which is initially formed may be visible as a radiolucent horizontal line till the age of two or may even persist. There may then be a problem in distinguishing such a persisting C1-C2 disk from a fracture of the odontoid process [54, 57].

The axis is distinguished by its odontoid process (dens) which articulates with the posterior aspect of the anterior arch of the atlas. The dens and the body of the axis are flanked by a pair of large oval joint facets that articulate with the inferior facets of the atlas.

The thoracic vertebrae increase in size from T1 to T12. They are distinguished by the presence of hemifacets on the lateral aspect of their bodies that articulate with the ribs. The ribs also articulate with the transverse processes. The long spinous processes slope steeply downward. Therefore, the axial section of a thoracic vertebral body still shows the spinous process of the vertebra above. The vertebral bodies have a larger anteroposterior than transverse diameter with a shallow concave posterior surface on the axial scan [43]. The spinal canal is round at the midthoracic level and rather triangular at the upper and lower ends.

The lumbar vertebrae are the largest. Their costal processes are frequently termed the transverse processes. However, they stem from the costal rudiment which fuses with the vertebra. The mamillary and accessory processes are the remainder of the true transverse process and are unique to the lumbar spine [52].

The pedicles, laminae and spinous processes are comparatively thick, encompassing the nearly triangular spinal canal [43]. The lateral recess is bounded anteriorly by the vertebral body and posteriorly by the pedicle and posterior arch.

The distribution of the bony trabeculae within the vertebra is not homogeneous. They are comparatively scarce in the anterior third of the vertebral body. This may contribute to the high number of impression wedge fractures.

The MR appearance of the vertebral column depends mainly on the signal from the bone marrow. Fat within the marrow of the vertebral bodies, neural arches and articular pillars has a fairly high signal in the T1-weighted images. Dense cortical bone surrounding these osseous structures virtually lacks signal [44].

II. Ligaments and Articulations

The intervertebral disks provide the primary connection between the vertebral bodies. They consist of two major components. The outer part, the anulus fibrosus, is comprised of fibrocartilaginous tissue and fuses with the bony end-plate of the adjacent vertebral bodies. The inner portion, the nucleus pulposus, is a remnant of the notochord and contains a mucoid material in which collagen fibers are embedded. Due to their elasticity, the intervertebral disks not only account for the spinal column's flexibility but also act as shock-absorbers.

The intervertebral disks are thinnest in the upper thoracic and thickest in the lumbar spine, their height ranging from 3 mm to 15 mm respectively. Accordingly, at axial CT the disks can be better imaged the more caudal they are. In cross-section, their shape and size conforms to the adjacent vertebrae with the exception of the cervical region, where in the lateral part the disk abuts against the uncinate processes. In CT, the healthy disk is homogeneous and denser than the adjacent thecal sac and epidural fat and even denser than the paravertebral musculature [43]. The density of the disks is about 50–110 HU [62]. Differentiation of the anulus fibrosus from the nucleus pulposus is not possible by CT.

On MRI the substance of the nucleus pulposus has a higher signal intensity than the surrounding fibrous tissue. This is especially prominent in T2-weighted images.

The anterior longitudinal ligament extends from the anterior tubercle of the atlas and from the basilar part of the occipital bone down to the sacrum. It is a long, broad fibrous band and runs along the anterior surfaces of the vertebral bodies to which it is firmly attached. However, there is no such tight connection with the disks [52, 82].

The posterior longitudinal ligament is located within the spinal canal dorsal to the vertebral bodies. It is the direct continuation of the membrana tectoria and courses along the posterior aspects of the vertebral bodies to the sacrum. Recent investigations have shown that it consists of two layers. The superficial layer has no connexion with the vertebrae. The deep layer shows a segmental arrangement. Its fibers radiate medially into the disks, caudally into the end-plates and more laterally into the pedicles and the caudal portion of the anulus [95]. At the lumbar midvertebral level, the posterior longitudinal ligament is occasionally seen on CT as a thin line immediately posterior to the retrovertebral plexuses, as it is separated from the midportions of the vertebral bodies by vascular and connective tissue structures [42].

The ligamenta flava have a strictly segmental arrangement. They are stretched between the neural arches and consist of elastic fibers which account for their yellowish colour. They act as an aid in erection of the trunk.

On CT the ligamenta flava have an intermediate density and are readily demonstrated inferior and anterior to the laminae at the dorsal aspect of the spinal canal. They can be traced laterally into the neural foramina [42].

The interspinous ligaments are short segmental fibrous bands, extending between the spinous processes of neighboring vertebrae. Their orientation is in an oblique direction, as they extend from the tip of one spinous process to the base of the next lower one. Thus, they are not only an obstacle to excessive flexion, but also prevent dorsal slipping of the vertebra above.

Ligaments can be delineated best either by CT or MRI when they are surrounded by their natural contrast medium, fat. This is constantly true for the ligamenta flava. On MRI it is often impossible to distinguish between the low-intensity ligamentous structures, the dura, anulus fibrosus and adjacent cortical bone of the vertebral body [80].

The interspinous and supraspinous ligaments may show gaps at certain levels. Circumscribed loss of visualization is therefore no proof of rupture.

The inferior articular processes of the upper vertebra and the superior articular process of the lower vertebra articulate by the zygapophyseal joints, diarthrodial articulations in which the articular process of the superior vertebra lies posterior to its lower vertebrae counterpart. Each articular surface is covered with cartilage. The joint space is covered by an articular capsule which is rather loose in the cervical spine and rather tight in the lumbar spine. The neural foramen is located immediately anterior to the facet joint.

At the craniocervical junction, the ligamentous and articular anatomy is rather complex.

The atlantoaxial articulations comprise four synovial joints: The median ones in front and back of the odontoid process and the lateral zygapophyseal joints. The anterior median atlantoaxial joint is situated between the anterior surface of the dens and the posterior surface of the anterior arch of the atlas. The posterior joint lies between the cartilage-covered anterior surface of the transverse ligament and the posterior surface of the dens.

The atlas and axis are connected by the cruciform and anterior and posterior longitudinal ligaments and by the articular capsules. The transverse part of the cruciate ligament, the transverse ligament, arches across the ring of the atlas behind the dens. At either end it is attached to a tubercle at the inner aspect of the lateral mass of the atlas. It prevents atlantoaxial dislocation. Rupture of this strong ligament has similar consequences as fracture of the odontoid process.

Of the craniocervical ligaments the tectorial membrane, the anterior and posterior atlanto-occipital membranes and the apical ligament should be mentioned. The alar ligaments are two strong bands that arise at each end of the upper part of the dens and extend obliquely upward and outward to attach to the medial surface of the occipital condyles. Axial rotation of the craniocervical junction is limited by these ligaments.

On axial CT, the transverse ligament appears as a thick regular stripe, concave forward around the posterior aspect of the dens and prominent with its marked hyperdensity [11]. Laterally, its fibrous bundles fan out to reach the tubercles of the atlas. On axially oriented MRI slices the transverse ligament is identified as a low signal intensity structure. The alar ligaments are poorly demonstrated on axial slices. Coronal CT or MRI sections are required to show them in their entirety.

III. Spinal Cord and Meninges

The spinal cord in general is a cylinder of nervous tissue contained within the spinal canal. After the first trimester of embryonic development, the vertebral column grows faster than the cord, with the result that the adult spinal cord ends approximately at the upper border of the second lumbar vertebra. The cord has two major enlargements: the cervical enlargement (C3 to T2) and the lumbar enlargement (T9 to L2) mark the origin of the nerves of the brachial and lumbosacral plexuses.

The spinal cord terminates in the conus medullaris. At the conus, the filum terminale arises from the cord and attaches it to the dorsal aspect of the coccyx.

The gray matter of the spinal cord is located centrally around the central canal. In cross-section it is "H"- or butterfly-shaped with anterior, lateral and posterior horns. The anterior horn of the gray matter represents an aggregation of cell bodies of the motor nerves known as the anterior horn cells. The white matter in turn contains bundles of nerve fibers which are distributed as funiculi (anterior, lateral and posterior) around the gray matter.

The anterior median fissure of the spinal cord is deep and contains a fold of pia mater. It is best visualized on CT myelography or on transverse MR slices.

On axial CT, the spinal cord appears as a homogeneous elliptical structure with a slightly higher signal intensity than CSF. Thus, it can be delineated on unenhanced CT scans only when surrounded by a sufficiently thick band of CSF. The cord is often not discriminated in routine unenhanced images [42], especially in the thoracic spine where the subarachnoid space is narrowest.

The spinal cord is best visualized on sagittal MR scans. The diameter of the cord increases slightly from the level of the third cervical to the second thoracic vertebra and from the ninth thoracic to the second lumbar vertebra where the roots of the brachial and lumbar plexuses arise. Though axial MR sections and certain pulse sequences are able to discriminate white from gray cord substance, differentiation of the individual tracts and funiculi is not possible on either CT or MR scans [44].

The central canal, a continuation of the ventricular system, is a small ependyma-lined space located in the gray matter and extending throughout the spinal cord. Thin sagittal MR sections occasionally show the central canal, but this may be difficult to distinguish from artifacts.

A pair of spinal nerves, 31 in all, arise from the spinal cord at every level and exit through the corresponding intervertebral foramen. Each nerve is composed of an anterior motor and a posterior sensory root. Each dorsal sensory root forms the dorsal root ganglion at the level of the intervertebral or neural foramen. Distal to the dorsal root ganglion the posterior and anterior root fuse to form a mixed spinal nerve. The spinal nerves exit through the neural foramina with a dural sleeve designated as the root-sheath. These sheaths are surrounded by fat.

The neural foramen contains fat, part of the ligamentum flavum, a meningeal nerve sheath with the anterior and posterior root, the spinal ganglion and some tiny vessels. On CT the spinal nerve roots are readily distinguished as soft tissue structures embedded in the epidural fat. The nerve root ganglion is visible as an enlargement in the lateral nerve root sheath. Intrathecal contrast medium opacifies the sheath proximal to the ganglion; lateral to it, the slender nerve silhouette can be traced for a few centimeters [42]. In T1-weighted MR images, the root-sheaths containing the nerve roots can be distinguished as low signal structures [44].

There are 12 thoracic, 5 lumbar, 5 sacral and 1 coccygeal spinal nerves, each of them exiting the vertebral canal immediately below the corresponding vertebra. On the other hand, in the cervical region the spinal nerves exit the spinal canal above the corresponding vertebra. This leaves one spinal nerve, C8, which exits below C7 and above T1.

The difference in growth rate between the spinal cord and spinal column explains why spinal cord segments are located above their corresponding vertebral levels. The lower the cord segment, the longer the distance between the origin of the root from the cord and its exit from the spinal column.

The spinal roots of the lumbar and sacral segments travel a long distance through the spinal canal where they resemble a horse's tail. This explains for their anatomic name of "cauda equina".

The spinal cord is surrounded by three membranes, the meninges. The dura mater is the outermost. The dural sac extends from the occiput to the sacrum and is normally seen on CT as a smooth slightly hyperdense layer separating its hypodense aqueous contents from the epidural fat. The pia mater, the innermost membrane, covers the surface of the spinal cord. Between the dura and pia mater lies the arachnoid.

The epidural space separates the dural sac from the vertebral column. Besides fat, it mainly contains venous plexuses. The subdural space separates the dura mater from the arachnoid membranes and the subarachnoid space separates the arachnoid webs from the pia mater. Cerebrospinal fluid is contained within the subarachnoid space. In the subarachnoid space, the delicate denticulate ligament connects the lateral aspect of the cord with the dural sac.

The subarachnoid space is seen on CT as a hypodense layer surrounding the cord substance or the hypodense contents of the lumbar spinal canal, which comprise the CSF and the cauda equina. On MRI the appearance of the CSF depends on the pulse sequence selected and on possible artifacts. The nerve-roots and the cauda equina traversing the subarachnoid space are best assessed on CT after injection of intrathecal contrast medium. Thin-section MR is also capable of depicting these structures.

The epidural space is identified on CT by its hypodense fat-equivalent density. Tiny soft tissue structures correspond with epidural vessels and nervous structures. On MRI the epidural fatty tissue is prominent by virtue of its short T1 values. Its vascular components have a low signal in most sequences. With intravenous administration of a paramagnetic contrast medium, however, a bright signal is obtained from the venous plexuses on T1-weighted pulse sequences [44]. The epidural space is most prominent at the upper and mid-thoracic spine.

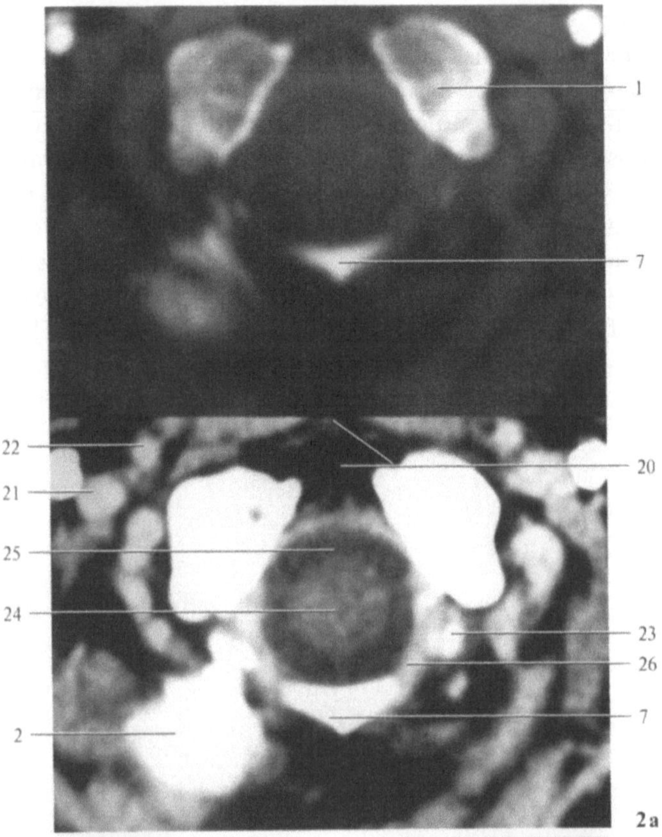

2a

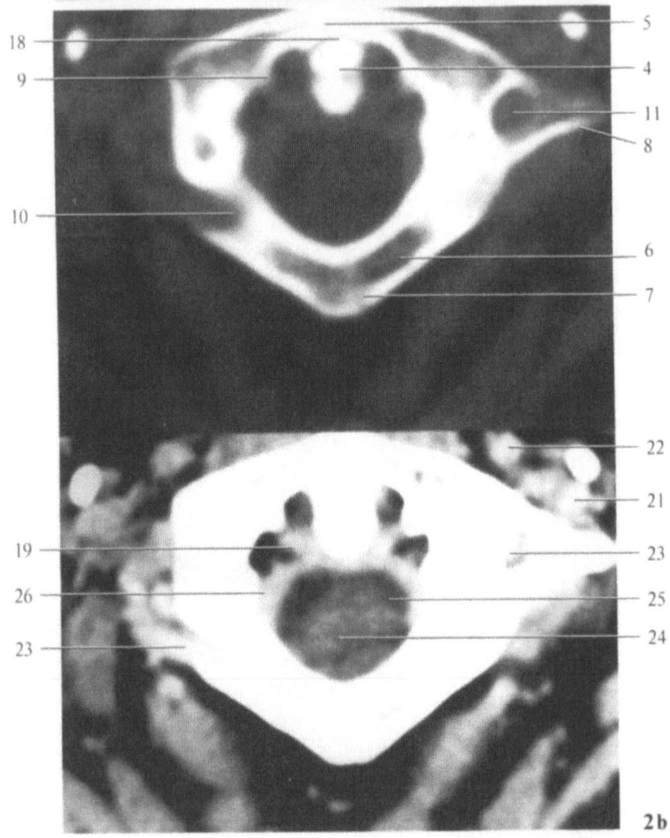

2b

Fig. 2 a–d. CT of the craniocervical junction. **a–c** Axial, **d** coronal section after i. v. injection of contrast medium

1 Occipital condyle
2 Occipital bone
3 Jugular foramen
4 Odontoid process (dens)
5 Anterior arch of C1
6 Posterior arch of C1
7 Posterior tubercle of C1
8 Transverse process of C1
9 Lateral mass of C1
10 Groove for vertebral artery
11 Foramen of the transverse process ("transverse foramen") of C1
12 Inferior articular facet of C1
13 Superior articular facet of C2
14 Spinous process of C2
15 Body of C2
16 Atlanto-occipital joint
17 Lateral atlanto-axial joint
18 Median atlanto-axial joint
19 Transverse ligament
20 Anterior atlanto-occipital membrane
21 Internal jugular vein
22 Internal carotid artery
23 Vertebral artery
24 Spinal cord
25 Subarachnoid space
26 Epidural space with venous plexus
27 Posterior cranial fossa

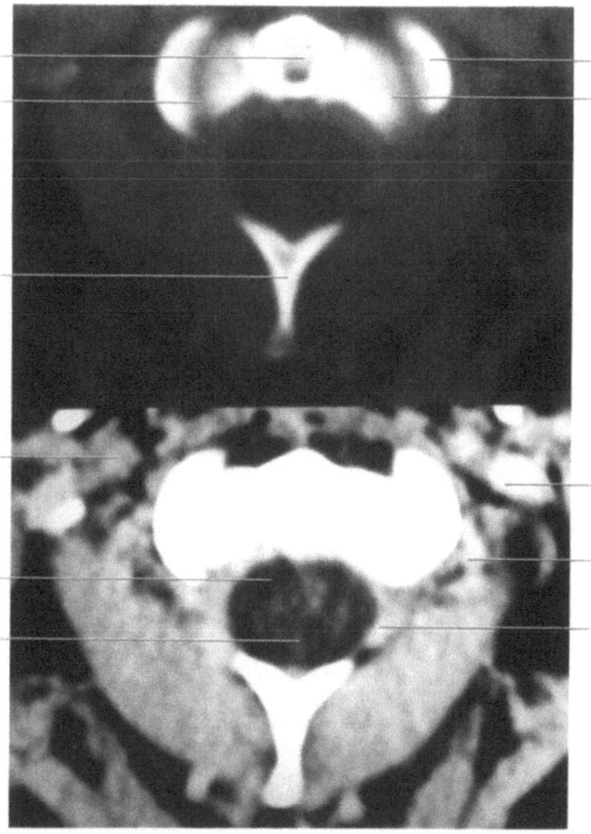

2c

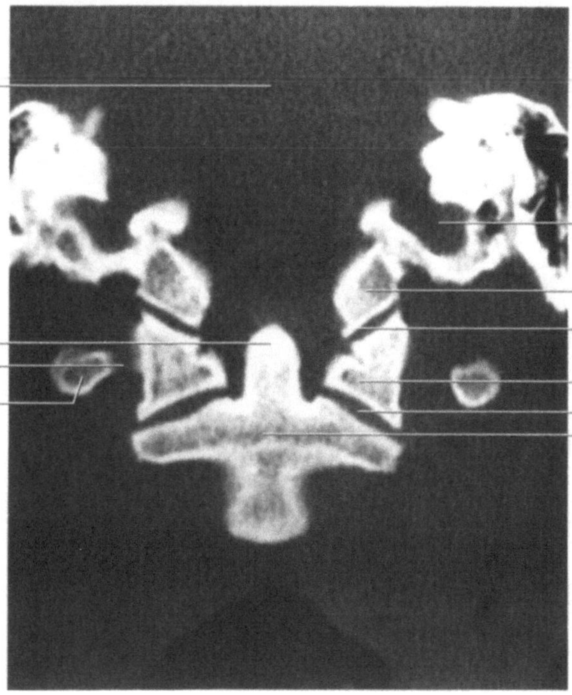

2d

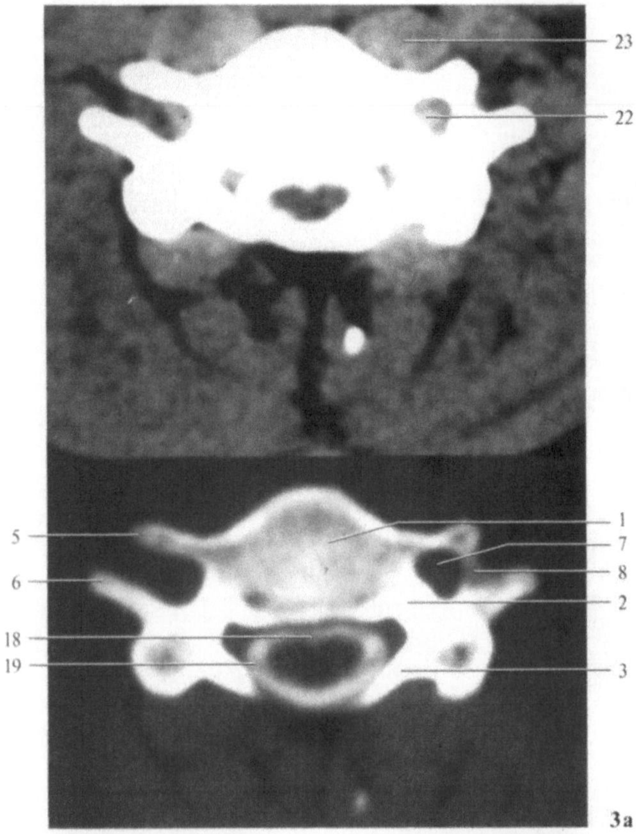

3a

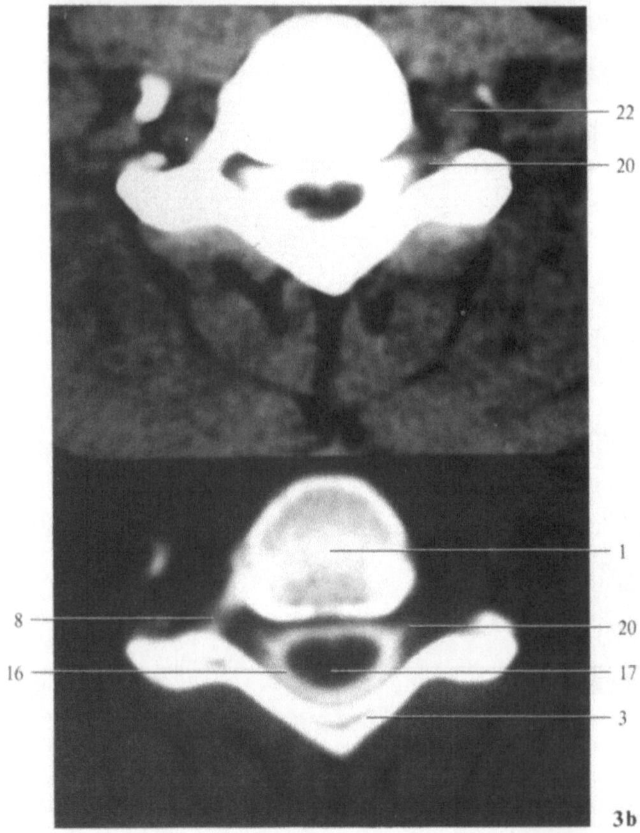

3b

Fig. 3. a–d Axial CT myelography sections at C4/C5 level from cranial to caudal

1 Vertebral body of C4
2 Pedicle
3 Lamina
4 Transverse process
5 Anterior tubercle
6 Posterior tubercle
7 Foramen of the transverse process ("transverse foramen")
8 Sulcus of the spinal nerve
9 Spinous process of C4
10 Uncinate process of C5
11 Intervertebral foramen C4/C5
12 Inferior articular process of C4
13 Superior articular process of C5
14 Zygoapophyseal joint
15 Epidural space
16 Subarachnoid space
17 Spinal cord
18 Anterior root of C5
19 Posterior root of C5
20 Root sheath
21 Dorsal root ganglion
22 Vertebral artery
23 Longus colli muscle
24 Intervertebral disk
25 Uncovertebral joint

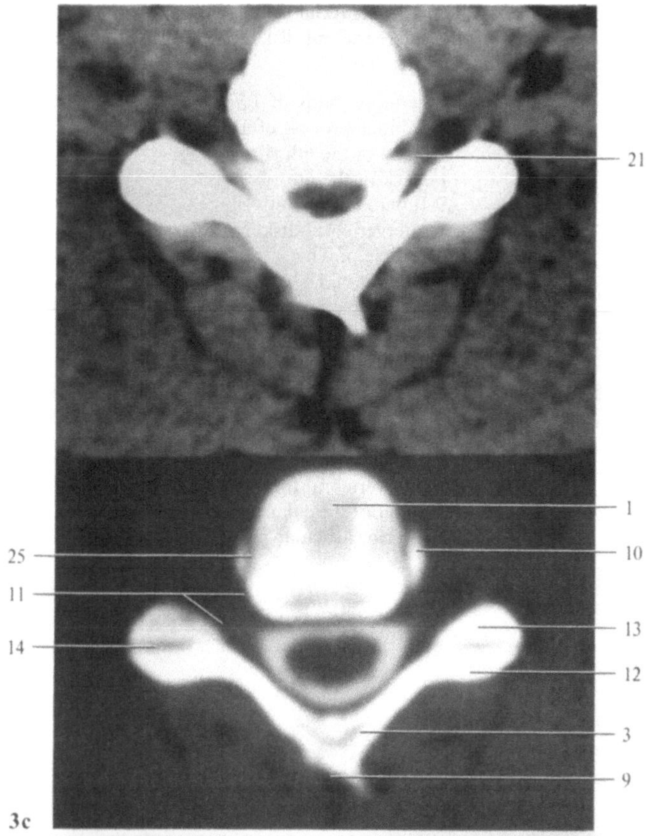

3c

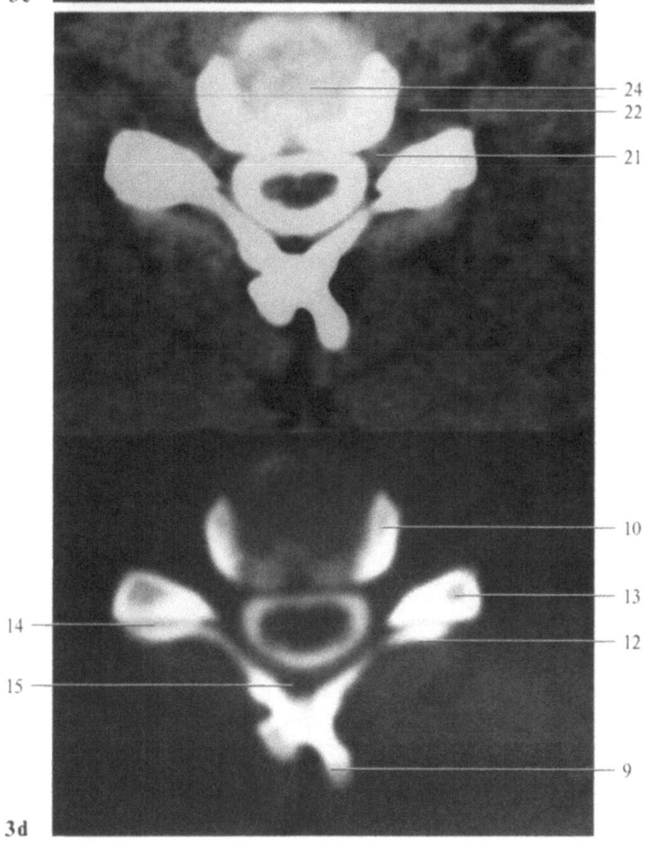

3d

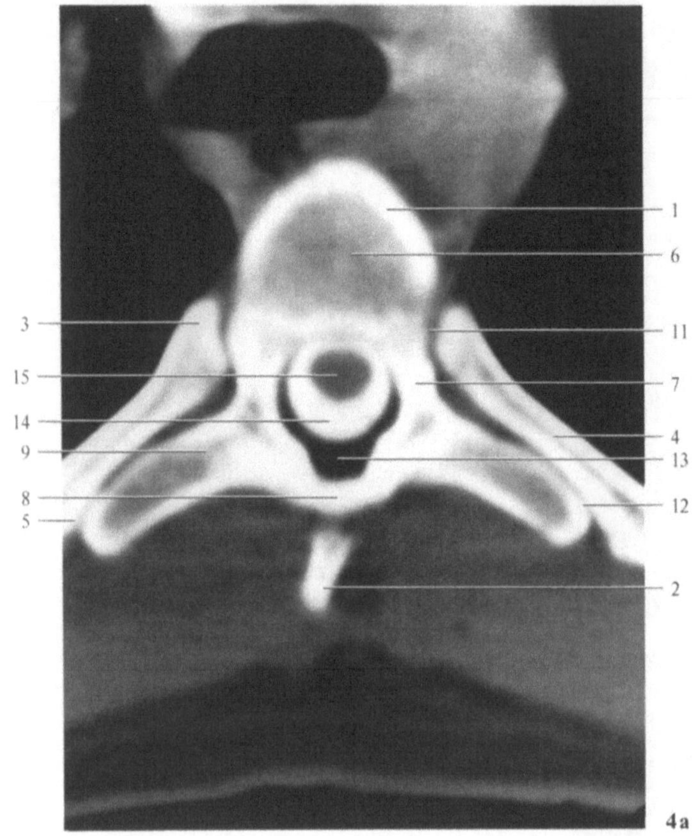

Fig. 4 a, b. Axial CT myelography. **a** At the level of the intervertebral disk T5/T6. **b** At the intervertebral foramen T6/T7

1 Vertebral body of T5
2 Spinous process of T5
3 Head of the 6th rib
4 Neck of the 6th rib
5 Tubercle of the 6th rib
6 Intervertebral disk T5/T6
7 Pedicle of T6
8 Lamina of T6
9 Transverse process of T6
10 Vertebral body of T6
11 Costovertebral joint of T6
12 Costotransverse joint of T6
13 Epidural space
14 Subarachnoid space
15 Spinal cord
16 Intervertebral foramen T6/T7
17 Superior articular process of T7
18 Inferior articular process of T6

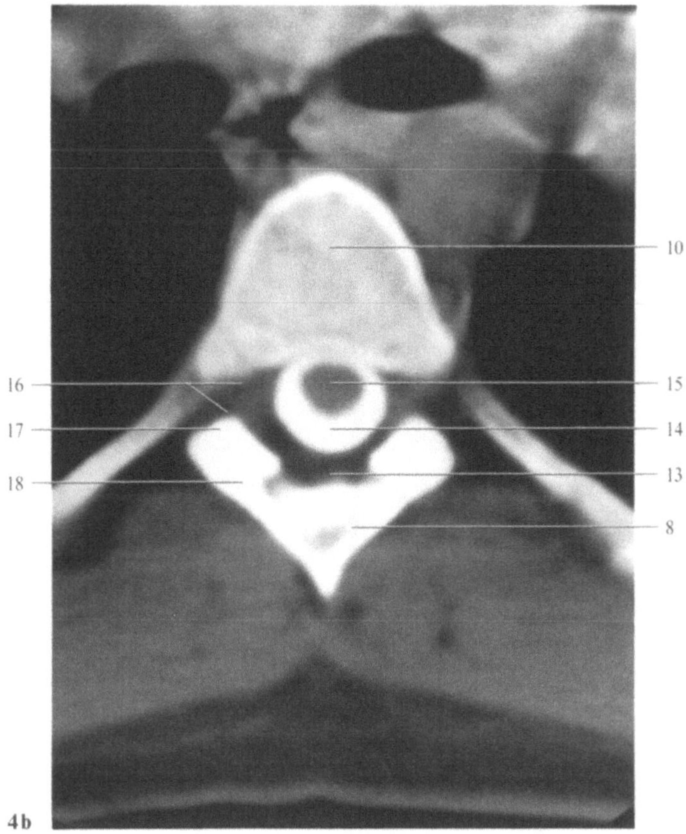

4b

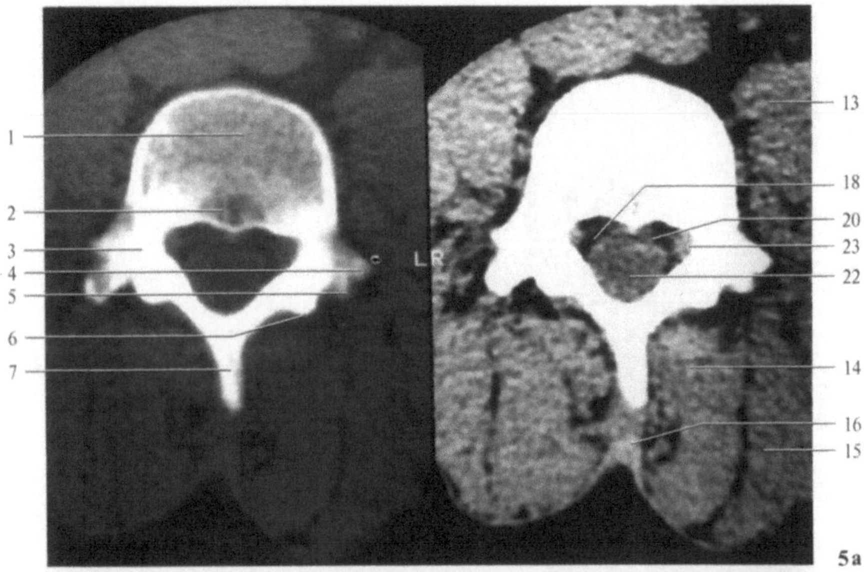
1
2
3
4
5
6
7
L R
13
18
20
23
22
14
16
15

5a

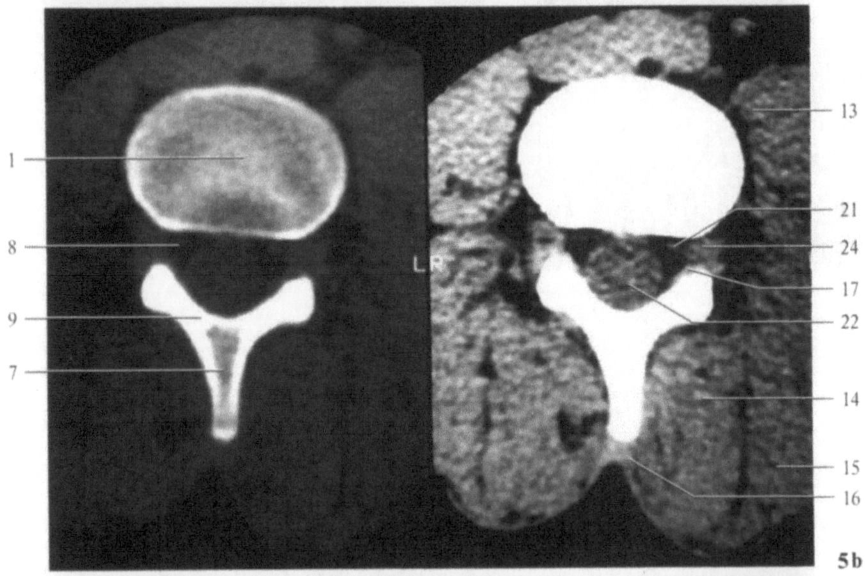
1
8
9
7
L R
13
21
24
17
22
14
15
16

5b

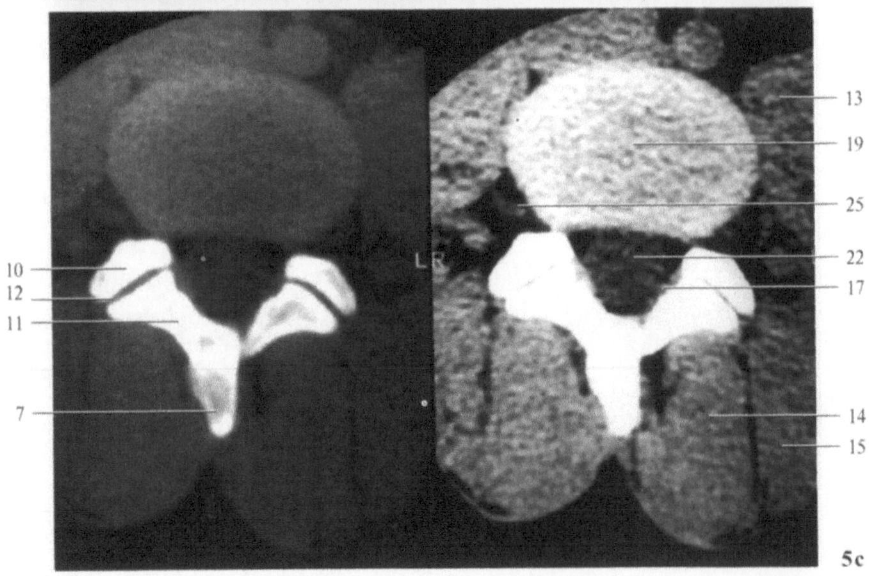
10
12
11
7
L R
13
19
25
22
17
14
15

5c

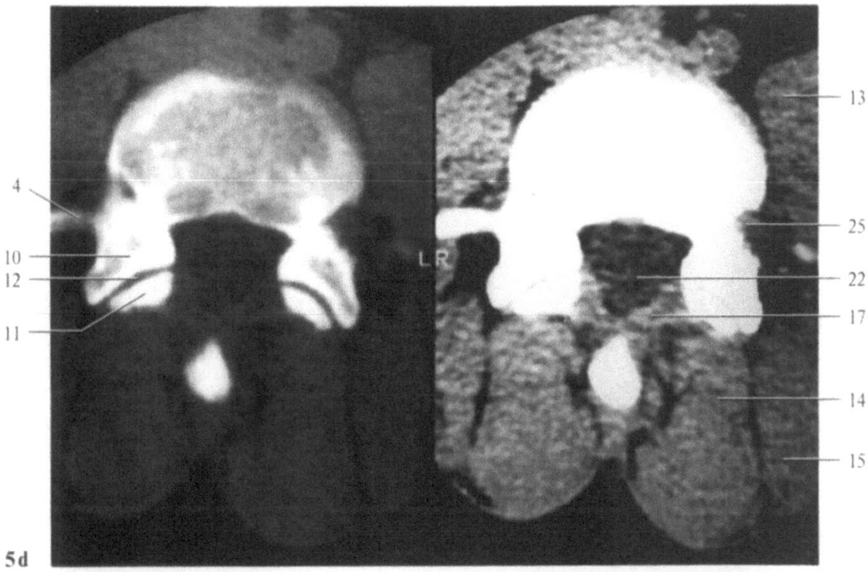

5d

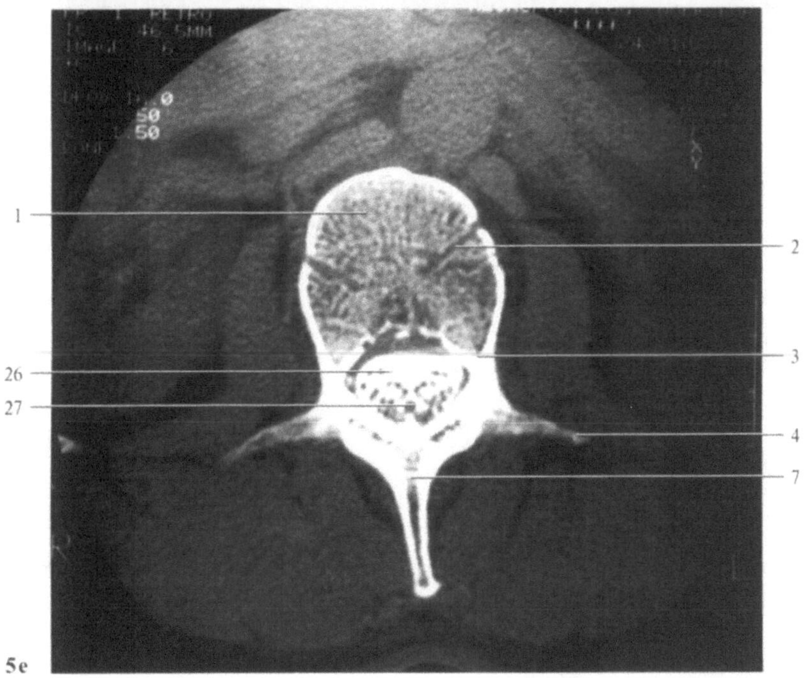

5e

Fig. 5. a–d Consecutive axial CT sections at the L4/L5 level from cranial to caudal. **e** Axial CT myelography of the 2nd lumbar vertebra

1 Vertebral body
2 Channel of the basivertebral vein
3 Pedicle
4 Costal process
5 Accessory process
6 Mamillary process
7 Spinous process
8 Intervertebral foramen
9 Lamina
10 Superior articular process
11 Inferior articular process
12 Zygoapophyseal joint
13 Psoas muscle
14 Multifidus muscle
15 Erector spinae muscle
16 Supraspinous and interspinous ligaments
17 Ligamentum flavum
18 Epidural fat
19 Intervertebral disk
20 Anterior internal vertebral venous plexus
21 Radicular vein
22 Thecal sac
23 Nerve root
24 Dorsal root ganglion
25 Spinal nerve
26 Cauda equina
27 Filum terminale

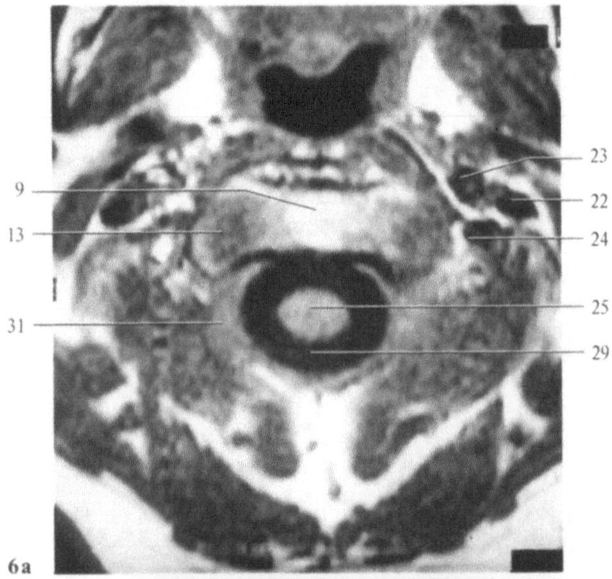
9
13
31
23
22
24
25
29

6a

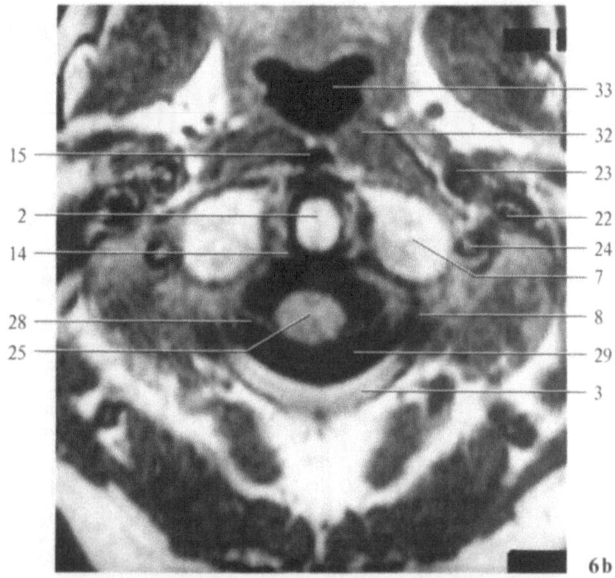
15
2
14
28
25
33
32
23
22
24
7
8
29
3

6b

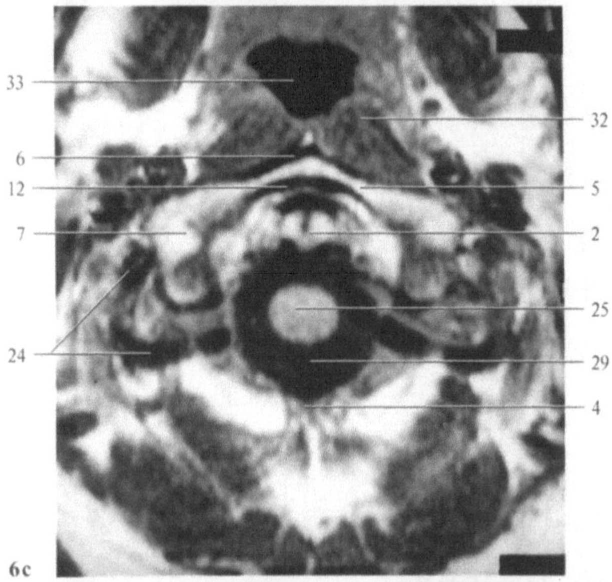
33
6
12
7
24
32
5
2
25
29
4

6c

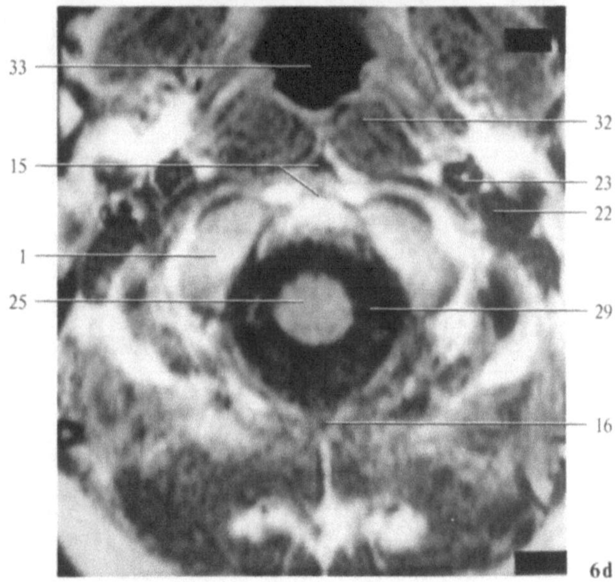
33
15
1
25
32
23
22
29
16

6d

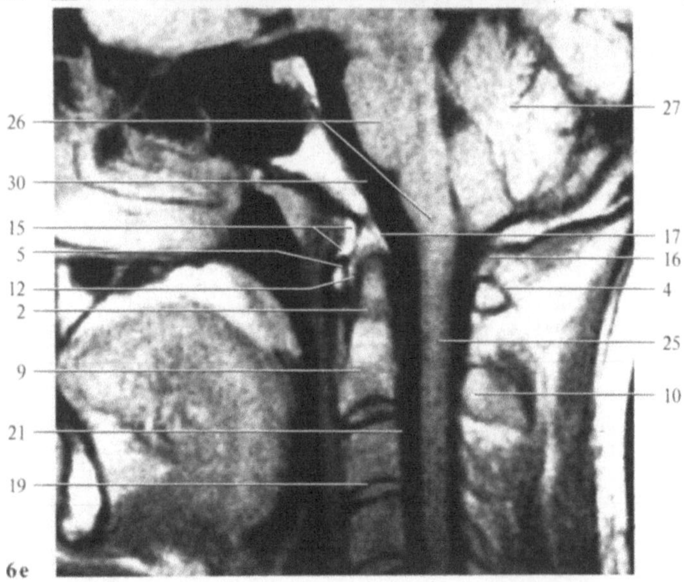
26
30
15
5
12
2
9
21
19
27
17
16
4
25
10

6e

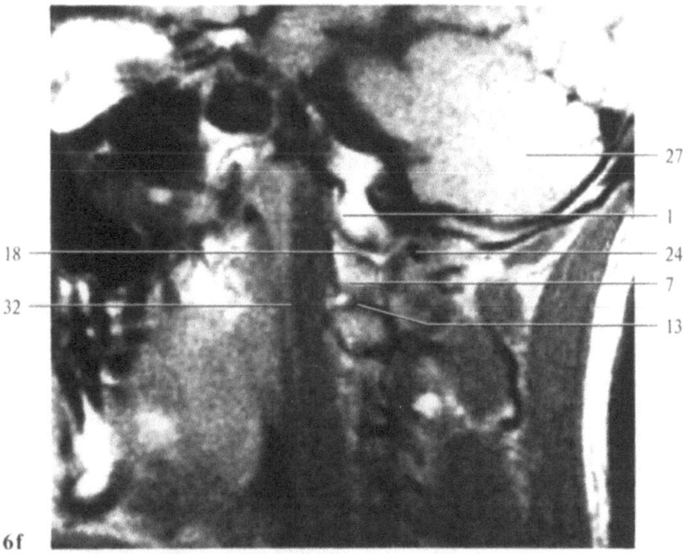

6f

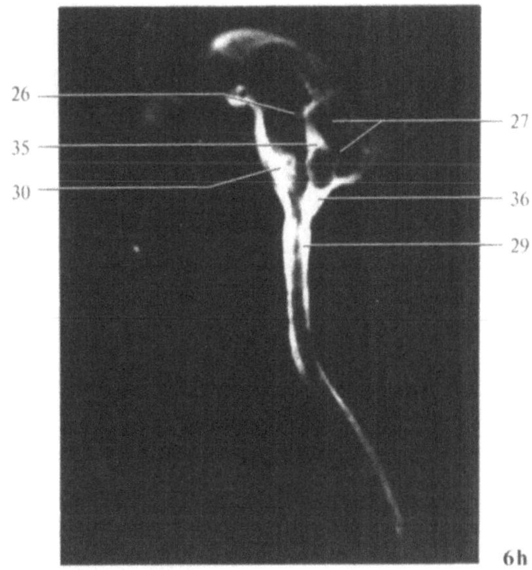

6h

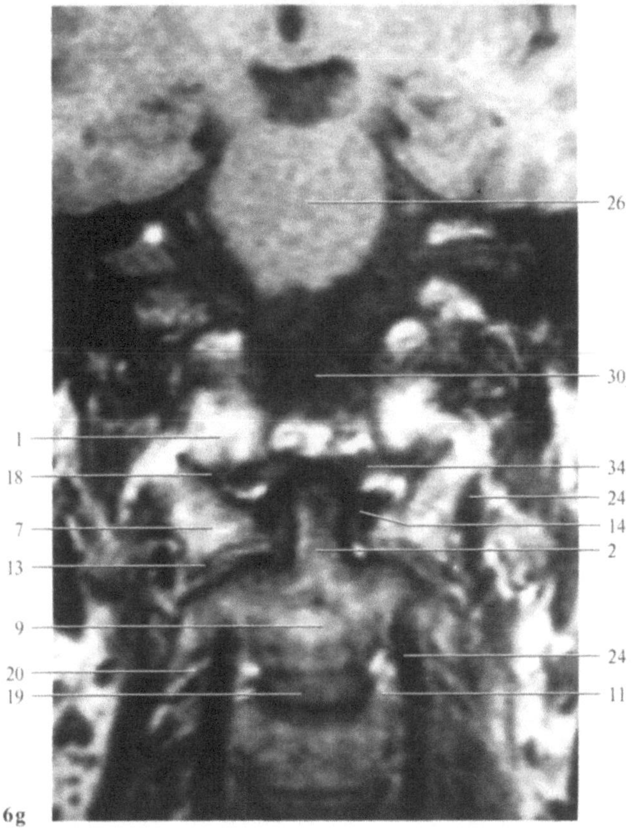

6g

Fig. 6 a–h. MRI of craniocervical junction. **a–d** Axial views (T1-weighted). **e–f** Sagittal slices (T1-weighted). **g** Coronal section (T1-weighted). **h** Sagittal MR-Myelography (extremely T2-weighted)

1 Occipital condyle
2 Odontoid process
3 Posterior arch of C1
4 Posterior tubercle of C1
5 Anterior arch of C1
6 Anterior tubercle of C1
7 Lateral mass of C1
8 Groove for vertebral artery
9 Body of C2
10 Spinous process of C2
11 Uncinate process
12 Median atlanto-axial joint
13 Lateral atlanto-axial joint
14 Transverse ligament
15 Anterior atlanto-occipital membrane
16 Posterior atlanto-occipital membrane
17 Apical ligament of the dens
18 Atlanto-occipital joint
19 Intervertebral disk
20 Zygoapophyseal joint
21 Posterior longitudinal ligament, dura and compact bone
22 Internal jugular vein
23 Internal carotid artery
24 Vertebral artery
25 Spinal cord
26 Brain stem
27 Cerebellum
28 Posterior root of C1 spinal nerve
29 Subarachnoid space
30 Ponto-medullary cistern
31 Epidural space with venous plexus
32 Longus colli and capitis muscle
33 Epipharynx
34 Alar ligament
35 4th ventricle
36 Cerebello-medullary cistern

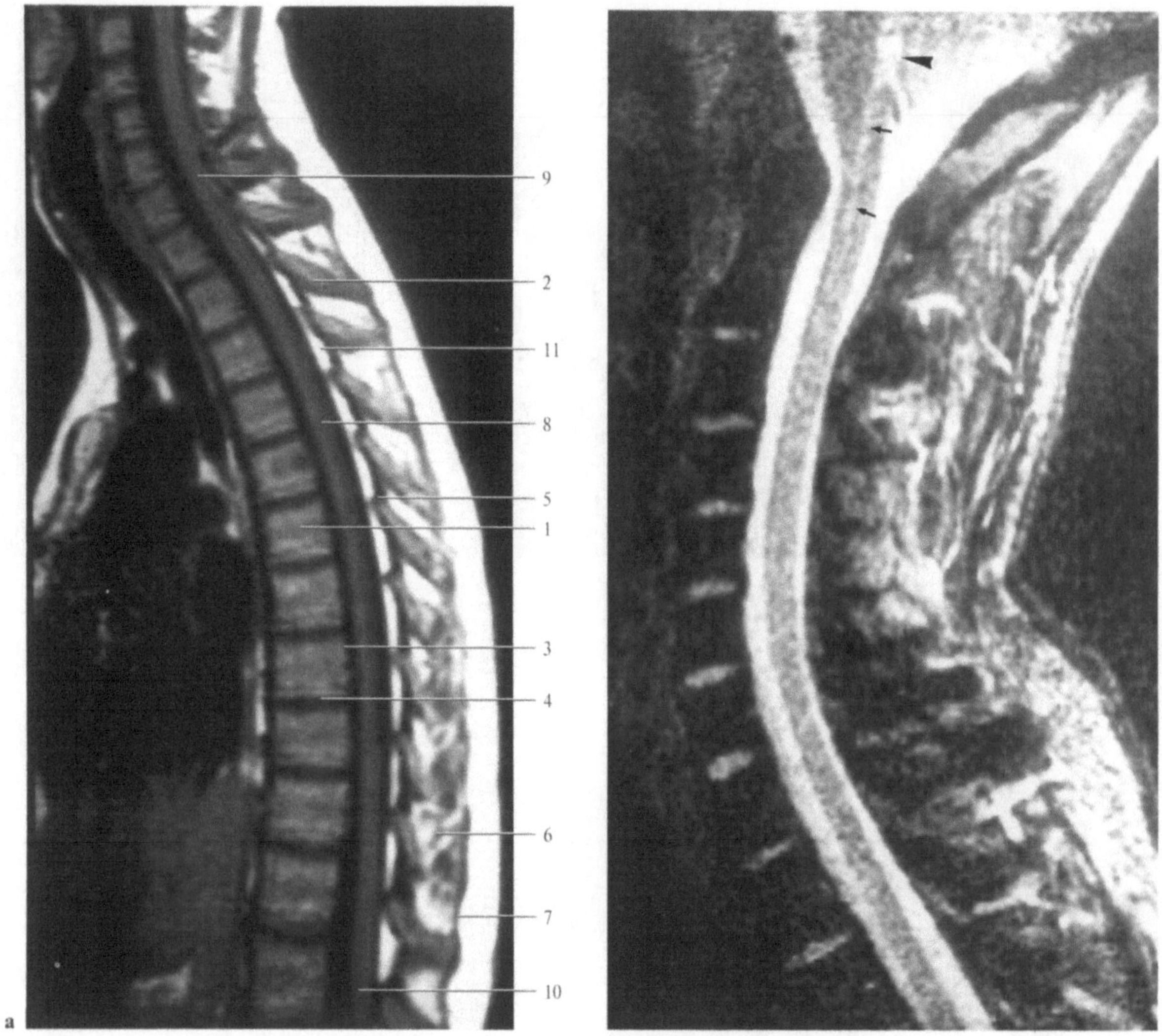

Fig. 7 a, b. Midsagittal MR section of the spine. **a** T1-weighted image. **b** T2-weighted image. The central canal *(arrows)* can be traced as a delicate hyperintense line from the fourth ventricle *(arrowhead)* to the spinal cord

1 Vertebral body
2 Spinous process
3 Cortical bone, posterior longitudinal ligament and dura
4 Intervertebral disk
5 Ligamentum flavum
6 Interspinous ligament
7 Supraspinous ligament
8 Spinal cord
9 Cervical enlargement
10 Lumbar enlargement
11 Epidural fat

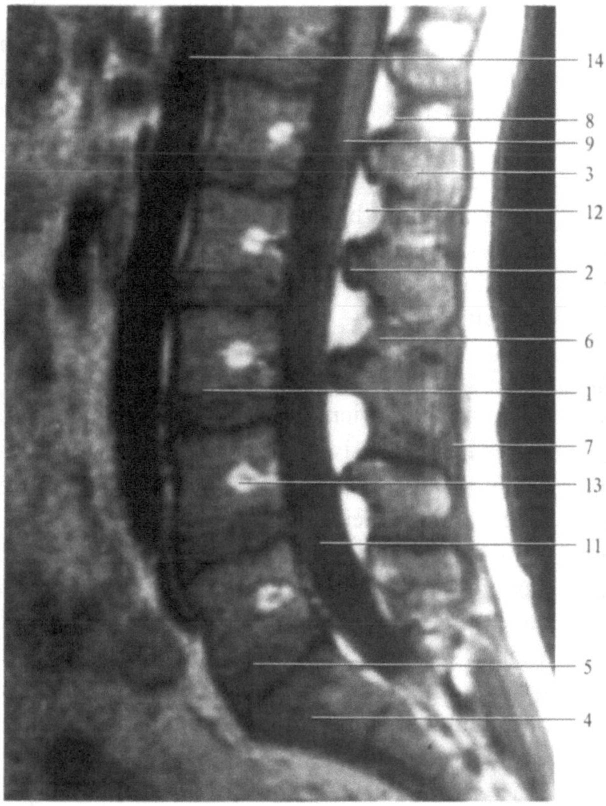

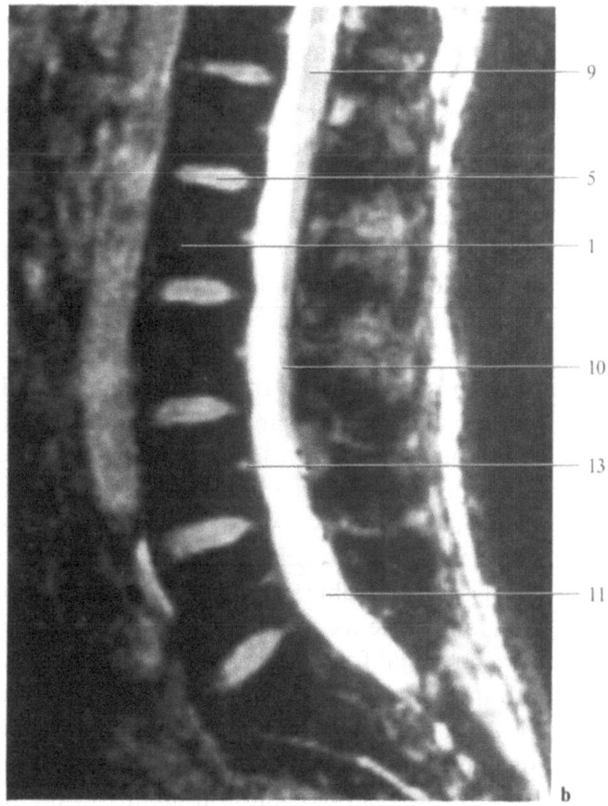

Fig. 8 a, b. MR of the lumbar spine. **a** T1-weighted midsagittal slice. **b** T2-weighted midsagittal cut

1 Vertebral body
2 Lamina
3 Spinous process
4 Sacrum
5 Intervertebral disk
6 Interspinous ligament
7 Supraspinous ligament
8 Ligamentum flavum
9 Conus terminalis
10 Cauda equina
11 Thecal sac
12 Epidural fat
13 Basivertebral vein
14 Abdominal aorta

C. Biomechanical Aspects, Stability and Fracture Classification

The most important and most difficult problem facing the diagnostician in the case of spinal fracture is the mechanical stability or biomechanics of the injured vertebral column. The answer is difficult enough even with a knowledge of spinal mechanics, and impossible without it. Modern imaging techniques make a decisive contribution here.

A consistent theory of the mechanics of the normal and injured spinal column does not yet exist, but some approaches thereto have been published particularly by WHITE and PANJABI [84, 91, 115] and by FARFAN and GRACOVETZKY [29, 35-37]. *Clinical Biomechanics of the Spine* [115] is a remarkable synopsis of current information, and since its appearance in 1978 the literature on spinal fractures has shown no significant advance. The glossary and the four chapters on physical properties and functional biomechanics, dynamics, the practical biomechanics of injury and the problem of clinical instability of the spinal column are recommended to those interested. We shall follow the intellectual structure of this work in our own short survey.

I. Some Physical Properties of the Elements of the Spine

1. Bony Structures

a) The Vertebral Body

The vertebral bodies may be considered as approximately cylindrical blocks of cancellous bone covered with a thin layer of cortical bone. Their size increases continuously in accordance with the increasing load from the first cervical vertebral body to the last lumbar body. The maximum axial load tolerance lies between around 1500 N at the third cervical vertebra and just 6000 N at the fifth lumbar body. After 40 years of age these threshold values become markedly lower.

About 55% of the load is borne by the cancellous bone of the vertebral body, and some 35% after the age of 40. A 25% loss of bony substance leads to a weakening of the vertebra by 50%. Together with the bone-marrow, the cancellous bone possesses shock absorbing properties in rapidly developing pressure loading of the spinal column. After a compression fracture it is often rigid, or even more rigid than an untraumatized bone, an observation that can be made on isolated cancellous blocks as well as on entire vertebral bodies [65, 89]. After loss of height by a half, the axial stability has again approximately its initial value.

b) The Articular Process

The variable orientation of the articular processes has a decisive influence on the nature and extent of the possible or "permissible" movements and on their coupling.

In the cervical spine the facet joints make an angle of some 45° to the horizontal, in the thoracic spine about 60° and in the lumbar spine about 90°. In addition, the joints in the thoracic spine are rotated by some 20° laterally and those of the lumbar spine some 45° medially, but there are marked individual differences.

This orientation results in the articular processes of the lumbar spine actively limiting rotation, whereas those of the thoracic spine impose no such restriction.

Hence, rotational rigidity increases steadily from the lower thoracic spine to the lumbar spine. Thus, it is nine times as great at L3-4 as at T7-8. There is an exception to this at the thoracolumbar junction, which exhibits the highest rotational rigidity, eleven times greater than T7-8. This sudden change in stability leads to a concentration of load and is one of the reasons for the striking frequency of fractures at the thoracolumbar junction.

The articular processes bear about a fifth of the axial load of the vertebral column. Sagittal flexion and especially extension are also effectively limited by intact articulations.

2. Disko-ligamentous Structures

Unlike the vertebrae, the ligaments of the spinal column and the intervertebral disks are bradytrophic structures. LOUIS points out that disko-ligamentous injuries therefore heal poorly, and that instability of ligamentous origin is therefore to be regarded as permanent [66].

a) The Intervertebral Disk

The intervertebral disk constitutes the primary connection between two vertebral bodies. It consists of the mucogelatinous nucleus pulposus and the anulus fibrosus composed of concentrically arranged fibrous layers. The fibers in the individual layers run parallel at an angle of $+30°$ or $-30°$ to the plane of the disk, thereby forming an angle of 120° from layer to layer. This arrangement is optimal for absorbing the centrifugal pressure which is mediated by a healthy nucleus pulposus in axial loading of the disk.

The inner layers are united with the cartilaginous end-plate of the vertebra; the outer layers are attached directly to the bone and are known as Sharpey's fibers. This latter connexion is substantially firmer.

The sum of the heights of all the disks amounts to a quarter to a third of the length of the vertebral column.

With increasing axial loading the healthy intervertebral disk is initially relatively compliant but then exhibits increasing resistance, its behavior resembling that of a shock-absorber with progressive characteristics. Under further loading there next occurs failure of the end-plate of the vertebral body and the formation of hernias of the nucleus pulposus into the cancellous bone. Experimentally, disk prolapse cannot be produced by axial pressure loading alone [73, 114]. The physiologic intradiscal intranuclear pressure was measured by NACHEMSON et al. [78] in vivo. In sitting or standing it amounts to double the whole body-weight, and becomes threefold if a weight of 20 kg is held in the hand.

The degeneratively altered intervertebral disk shows another characteristic. The dehydrated nucleus pulposus cannot absorb and deviate laterally any load. Hence the axial load is transmitted by the anulus fibrosus alone, so that the outer zones of the vertebral body are stressed relatively more than the center of the end-plate. Fractures of the outer zones of the end-plate therefore become more probable with increasing degeneration of the nucleus pulposus. The disk is less resistant to axial traction strain.

In flexion and extension there is bulging of the anulus fibrosus on the pressure side and retraction on the traction side. The disk is sensitive to torsion. FARFAN showed that small angles of up to around 3° can be produced by very small rotational forces. For angles between 3° and 20°, rotational force and resultant rotational angle increase in linear relationship. At about 20° or 30 Nm there is failure of the disk [28]. Shearing forces are tolerated, significantly better the resistance here being about a tenth of resistance to pressure. Destruction of the disk by purely shearing forces is therefore rather improbable; usually, they are combined with forward or lateral flexion or rotation.

b) The Ligaments

As in other joints, the ligaments of the spinal column limit the range of movement. They are only effective against traction strain. Within physiologic limits they oppose movements with only slight resistance, but this rises steeply at these bounds. They can absorb high acceleration forces in whole or part. NOYES et al. [81] showed in cruciate ligament specimens in the rhesus monkey that, with gradually increasing force, the ligaments avulse bone but are themselves torn with more rapid increase.

The anterior longitudinal ligament extends from the anterior margin of the foramen magnum on the anterior aspect of the vertebral column to the sacrum. It is attached to the margins of the vertebral bodies and limits extension. Its rupture load amounts to some 340 N, the preload to 1.8 N [112]. The posterior longitudinal ligament extends initially as the tectorial membrane from the ophisthion over the back of the dens and transverse ligament, and then on the back of the vertebral bodies to the sacrum. According to PRESTAR and PUTZ [94], it consists of a superficial continuous layer and a deep segmentally arranged layer. The latter enters into an intimate connection with the intervertebral disk, the upper margin of the vertebral body and, in the cervical spine, the lower margin of the vertebral body as well. The rupture load is 180 N, preload 3.0 N respectively.

The ligamenta flava connect the inferior anterior edge of the upper lamina with the superior posterior edge of the lower lamina. They owe their yellow color to their large content of elastic fibers. Their initial stress is very high: 18 N in young persons and 5 N in the aged. On the one hand, this prevents protrusion of the ligament into the spinal canal; on the other, it exerts a constant rest-compression on the disk with resulting basic stability.

The role of the other ligaments and the capsules of the small intervertebral joints has not been much studied, though it is certain that the joint capsules are important in restricting rotation and flexion.

3. The Motion Segment

The concept of the motion segment was introduced into the literature by JUNGHANNS [106]. It consists of two adjacent vertebrae together with the connecting ligamentous structures and constitutes the smallest functional entity of the spinal column. Its mechanical properties resemble those of the entire spine. Hence it serves as the preferred object of biomechanical research into the spine, and it is conventional to describe the movement of the cranial vertebra relative to the caudal vertebra. WHITE and PANJABI place the origin of a three-dimensional, right-angled coordinate system at the midpoint of the upper of the two vertebrae under consideration. The y-coordinate coincides with the axis of the vertebral column; the x-axis is at right angles to this in the frontal plane and the z-axis runs ventrodorsally [115].

Thus, every movement may be described as a combination of the six basic types of motion ("degrees of freedom"), namely longitudinal translation to and rotation around the three axes. As already mentioned, the possible movements are limited by a system of disko-ligamentous and bony structures. An important consequence of these anatomic determinants is the so-called coupling. Actually, there is no simple translation or rotation around one of the three spatial axes, but in each case a superimposition of different basic movements with a varying degree of expression of the components.

For example, an antero-posterior displacement in the thoracic spine is always associated with rotation around the (latero-lateral) x-axis. Rotation of a lumbar vertebra around the y-axis always leads to lateral flexion.

As no true circumduction is described during rotation, the rotational axis changes with time. There is what is called an "instantaneous axis of rotation (IAR)", intended to specify the momentary movement of a body in one plane. A similar concept for three-dimensional movements is that of the "helical axis of motion (HAM)", which reduces the movement to the helical translation and rotation along an axis constructed from the components of movement in the three planes of space.

Special attention must be paid to the craniocervical junction with its great range of movement, particularly the 47° of rotation at C1-2 which makes considerable demands on the flexibility of the vertebral artery. The relatively great sagittal range of movement at C5-6 may be responsible for the frequency of degenerative diseases at this level.

4. The Rib Cage

The ribs together with the sternum and muscles brace the spine, especially in rotation and flexion movements, in two ways: first, by means of the costovertebral joints and costotransverse ligaments and second, because of the high inertial moment of the thorax. The possible axial loading of the spine is thereby raised four-fold. On the other hand, an isolated spinal column without muscles and thorax can only bear about 20 N (2 kg) of axial load without permanent deviation from the rest position.

The supportive action of the rib cage is lost with defects in the longitudinal axis, as in sternotomy or multiple rib fractures. The costovertebral joint plays an important part for the individual motion segment if all the posterior elements - the posterior longitudinal ligament and part of the disk - are destroyed, when it alone prevents slipping of the affected vertebra.

5. The Muscles

The muscles can be divided into a pre- and postvertebral group. They control and stabilize the movement of the spine within the physiologic limits. They function actively by contraction and passively - like other non-contractile tissues - by resistance to elongation.

6. The Spinal Cord

The spinal cord lies centrally within the rigid bony spinal canal, which changes its shape, length and diameter with movement, and is suspended from the meninges and the denticulate ligaments. The subarachnoid space contains arachnoidal connective tissue fibers and cerebrospinal fluid; the epidural space contains fat and vascular plexuses for further padding.

It is capable of adjusting to the changing local conditions by elongation or shortening. This is achieved by means of a concertina folding and unfolding of the fibers of the cord, i. e., a property of the structure and not of the material.

II. Stability and Fracture Classification

The stability of the spinal fracture is very difficult to assess, and many attempts have been made to define it. It has been described as early [22], or late [45], mechanical or neurologic [22], clinical [29, 55] or musculoskeletal [22] instability. It has been divided into three degrees or instability [19], or the term has been used without clear definition [6, 17]. In this context, "early" means that the instability appears immediately after the accident, "late" that it develops progressively with time. A fracture is termed neurologically unstable if it has produced spinal and/or root symptoms. Mechanical or musculoskeletal instability refers to the reduced load capacity of the axial skeleton after injury. The catastrophe theory has been invoked for clarification [55] and precise radiologic criteria of a clinical instability have been provided [115].

According to FARFAN and GRACOVETZKY [29]: "(clinical) instability is that (symptomatic) condition, where, in the absence of new injury, a physiological load induces abnormally large deformations at the intervertebral joint". They particularly stress the difference between an unstable mechanical system, here the damaged motion segment, and the consequences, such as cord compression, which may be produced by this instability.

WHITE and PANJABI [115] give a similar definition: clinical instability is "the loss of the ability of the spine under physiological loads to maintain relationships between vertebrae in such a way that there is neither initial damage nor subsequent irritation to the spinal cord or nerve roots and, in addition, there is no development of incapacitating deformity or pain due to structural changes".

By physiological loads these authors mean those encountered during normal activity of the patient investigated. This means the abandonment of the concept of an absolute stability, defined in terms of the pathologic anatomy of the situation, and its replacement by a patient-related stability. The question is no longer whether an injured spinal column is stable *per se,* but whether it is sufficiently stable for a definite load in a definite direction. This seems to us the proper way to an individual assessment of the situation in a given patient. We therefore use the definition of FARFAN and GRACOVETZKY and interpret "physiological load" as do WHITE and PANJABI.

How then is this definition to be transferred to clinical practice?

A strategy for the patient in question must be evolved from consultation among the relevant diagnosticians and therapists, based on an exact description of the pathologic anatomy with a biomechanical assessment of the individual injury and mode of injury (e. g., compression/distraction), and with due attention to the clinical situation, the healing tendency of the affected tissue and the expected mechanical strains of the damaged spine.

Classifications are an adjunct to facilitate this task and simultaneously provide a common idiom for those engaged in diagnosis and treatment. Any classification should satisfy the following requirements:

It should be simple and easily remembered, it should not be dependent on the employment of sophisticated diagnostic methods, it should allow immediate interpretation, it should provide information about details and a guide to the best form of treatment, and it should give an indication of the prognosis [61].

Such classifications are not yet available for spinal fractures at the present time and are therefore, like stability, the subject of controversial debate. One initial and fundamental problem is the variable anatomy of the different parts of the spine. Most classifications therefore relate to particular spinal regions, usually the lower cervical spine or the thoracolumbar section.

Classifications exist in terms of the descriptive morphology or pathobiomechanics, as well as every intermediate form with and without assertions as to stability. Imaging techniques always play a decisive part, and the presumed mechanism of injury is often reconstructed from the radiographs.

Almost all authors refer to the classification proposed in 1970 by HOLDSWORTH [46] for fractures below C2, based on his great experience. HOLDSWORTH divides the spine into two columns, a load-bearing anterior column and the posterior ligament complex, on the integrity of which the stability of the spine depends. He lists five types of fractures:

1. wedge fracture,
2. fracture-dislocation,
3. extension fracture,
4. burst fracture,
5. shearing fracture.

Types 1 and 4 are stable, type 3 is stable in flexion, while types 2 and 5 are completely unstable.

WHITE and PANJABI [115] adopt the division into anterior and posterior elements, with the borderline behind the posterior longitudinal ligament. They deduce from experiments on isolated motion segments that stability is preserved as long as either all the anterior elements and one additional posterior element or all the posterior elements and one additional anterior element are intact.

DENIS et al. [19, 21] then postulated the "three column theory" of the spine and the derived classification of thoracolumbar fractures, which involves a very similar formulation. This divides the spinal column into three vertical, metamerically arranged sections.

The anterior column consists of the anterior longitudinal ligament and the anterior two-thirds of the vertebral body and intervertebral disk, the middle column of the posterior third of the disk, the remaining portion of the vertebral body with its posterior margin and the posterior longitudinal ligament. The posterior column is composed

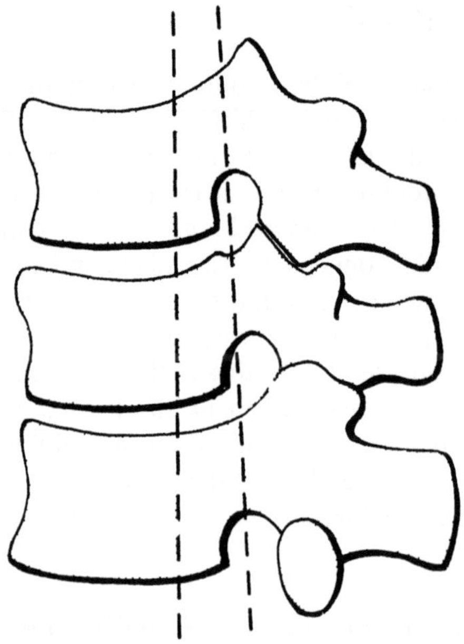

Fig. 9. The three column spine theory. Schematic drawing after DENIS and MCAFEE [19, 68]

of the posterior vertebral arch or bony complex in interplay with the ligamentous structures, i.e. the supraspinous and interspinous ligaments as well as the ligamenta flava and the articular capsules. These correspond to the "posterior ligamentous complex" of HOLDSWORTH.

DENIS regards it as essential that the middle column should remain intact, whereas the posterior column, like the medial collateral ligament of the knee-joint, plays only a modest role in the stability of a fracture.

This is the essential innovation compared with the hitherto widely accepted classification of HOLDSWORTH, from which it differs by regarding the complete burst fractures as unstable. If one pictures the development of a fracture, it is evident that this view is not basically different from that of WHITE and PANJABI. Injuries of the middle column are necessarily associated with (considerable) injuries of the anterior and/or posterior columns if direct injuries, as by gunshot wounds, are excluded. In a flexion fracture the middle column fails *after* the anterior column, and in an extension fracture *after* the posterior column, only if the energy exerted has not been expended in the destruction of the connected column. Rotational, translational and axial injuries are associated with injuries of all three columns. Thus, the destruction of the middle column is an index of a severe lesion of the spinal column. Conversely, integrity of the middle column also implies that the anterior and/or posterior columns are intact. This closely approximates to the requirement of PANJABI and WHITE already mentioned.

In his classification, DENIS initially divides the possible injuries of the spine into "major and minor spinal injuries". Interestingly, among minor injuries he includes not only fractures of the transverse and spinous processes as well as of the pars interarticularis, but also those of the articular processes, which LOUIS [66] regards as responsible for instability. HOLDSWORTH [46] also attributed great importance to them.

The major injuries are then divided into four main and 17 subcategories and the instability into three grades. This does not really seem very convenient for clinical practice, especially as no correspondingly different modes of treatment are available.

MCAFEE et al. [68] propose a simplified classification which bases its assessment on the forces acting on the middle column and the resulting pattern of injury. The three fundamental directions of force are axial compression, axial distraction and horizontal translation. This leads to subdivision into the following six groups:

1. wedge compression fracture with defect of the anterior column
2. stable burst fracture with defect of the anterior and middle columns from axial loading,
3. unstable burst fracture with additional defect of the posterior column,
4. Chance fracture as the outcome of axial traction which takes place through flexion around an axis in front of the vertebral body,
5. flexion-distraction injury with flexion around an axis dorsal to the anterior longitudinal ligament and a traction-induced defect of the middle and posterior columns,
6. translational injuries with the force exerted horizontally and disruption of the alignment of the spine.

MCAFEE [68] solves the problem of stability or instability of the burst fracture by making a distinction between stable and unstable burst fracture.

This classification was adapted essentially unchanged a little later by MAGERL [71] for German language usage. He translated "stable burst fracture" as "incomplete burst fracture" and "unstable burst fracture" as "complete burst fracture".

This led to therapeutic consequences. If the middle column is uninjured, no operative measures are usually necessary. The sole exception given by MCAFEE is the wedge fracture of several segments with a potentially progressive kyphosis. If the mechanism of injury was axial loading, treatment is by distraction; if it was caused by axial traction, compression is indicated. In translational injuries, compression - at least by HARRINGTON rods - is contraindicated.

FERGUSON and ALLEN [30] propose a so-called mechanistic classification, developed from some basic assumptions:

1. If part of a vertebral body is shortened, it must have undergone a compression force.
2. If part of a vertebral body is lengthened, a distraction force must have been applied.
3. Torsion forces produce rotational injuries of the affected segment.
4. Translational forces produce anterior, posterior or lateral displacements of the affected segment.

Thus, the pattern of injury makes it possible to infer the mechanism of injury and the groups are named correspondingly. The main categories are labelled:

1. compressive flexion,
2. distractive flexion,
3. lateral flexion,
4. translational,
5. torsional flexion,
6. vertical compression,
7. distractive extension.

Each of these is further subdivided into several stages of severity. These authors adopt the division of the spine into three anatomic regions, but reject the term "columns" as inappropriate.

For the lower cervical spine, ALLEN et al. [1] put forward a corresponding but slightly different system whose axioms are also varied. Their most important basic assumption is that the direction of the forces exerted ("injury vectors") may be derived from the plain film of the cervical spine. This concept, too, originates from WHITE and PANJABI who introduced the "major injury vector (MIV)" into the discussion.

In competition with the two above-mentioned classifications there is the point system proposed by LOUIS [66] in 1977, which has not become equally established in the English-language literature though its relative simplicity is agreeable to the user. It involves exclusively an assertion as to the stability or instability and is the only classification applicable to all sections of the spine, including the craniocervical junction.

LOUIS also distinguishes three osteoligamentous columns, but postulates one of these as the vertebral bodies and intervertebral disks in toto and the others as the two columns of the small vertebral articulations. These three columns form the vertical member of the two *"grands systèmes"*. The horizontal system is composed of the three "bony bridges" formed by both pedicles and both laminae. The transverse and spinous processes are regarded merely as lever arms for muscle attachments.

Each separate injury is allotted a point value: 1 for interruption of the continuity of one of the three vertical columns, 0.5 for fracture of one of the bony bridges and for incomplete transection of a vertical column, and finally 0.25 for the spinous and transverse processes as a whole.

The sum of these point values is the *"coéfficient d'instabilité"*. Increasing instability is indicated from a value of 2, while a value of 3 corresponds for instance to a complete dislocation. In marked contrast to MCAFEE, his assessment of fracture of a joint facet is double that of a pedicle fracture. This seems reasonable in view of the arguments advanced above for the special importance of the vertebral joints for rotational stability. LOUIS further refers to the different nature of bony and ligamentous instability. Bony instability is transient, but ligamentous instability is permanent because of the poor healing tendency of the affected bradytrophic tissue.

As already stated, the lower cervical spine occupies a special position as regards classification and assessment of stability. There are many individual descriptions of special types of fractures, such as the "tear-drop" fracture for example.

Table 4. Clinical instability of the lower cervical spine

Element	Point value
Anterior elements destroyed or unable to function	2
Posterior elements destroyed or unable to function	2
Relative sagittal plane translation >3.5 mm	2
Relative sagittal plane rotation >11°	2
Positive stretch test	2
Spinal cord damage	2
Nerve root damage	1
Abnormal disk narrowing	1
Dangerous loading anticipated	1

Total of 5 or more = unstable. WHITE and PANJABI [115, p 223]

ALLEN et al. [1] have provided a new and comprehensive classification for the lower cervical spine, as already set out above. It is attractive because of the clear deduction of fracture classes from the above-mentioned axioms. We share the authors' rejection of the "tear-drop" fracture and other vaguely defined concepts. Of course, we consider the classification as too extensive in its detail (6 groups and 21 grades). It represents an attempt to portray every injury as accurately as possible, and thereby differs only slightly from an individual description. The conventional radiologic criteria of each grade or stage are accurately described, but without use of the terms "stability" or "instability", and in our view this can only limit the making of therapeutic decisions. To be sure, the authors find a good correlation of the fracture grade with the severity of the neurologic features.

We therefore relinquish the idea of a classification of fractures of the lower cervical spine and limit ourselves to a statement as to stability. Here the point scores of LOUIS or WHITE are very helpful (Table 4).

1. Conclusion

The first task of the radiologist is to depict the pathologic anatomy accurately by imaging techniques. This is the prerequisite for an analysis leading to diagnosis.

The following statements seem permissible and reasonable:

1. The deformation illustrated by imaging techniques provides information as to the main force exerted, the major injury vector.
2. Analysis of the pathologic anatomy combined with functional views permits a statement on persisting mechanical stability against particular forces.
3. Indications for treatment can be derived therefrom.
4. Subject to limitations, the pattern of injury and the stability also indicate the prognosis.
5. The use of a classification is reasonable as a uniform mode of expression, at least within a clinic, and as an aid to documentation. Without clinical investigation of the patient and a detailed analysis of the damaged structures, it is inadequate for the choice of treatment.

D. Neurologic Symptoms in Spinal Trauma

Almost 20% of all injuries to the spinal column are associated with lesions of the spinal cord [64]. In 25% of vertebral fractures, neurologic deficits are encountered [105]. The areas of greatest mobility of the spinal column coincide with the most frequent sites of injury. Over a half of complete spinal cord injuries result in quadriplegia, often at the mid-cervical and lower cervical levels; less than half result in paraplegia, with injury most often at the thoracolumbar junction. The majority of spinal column injuries occur without any neurologic deficit.

I. Spinal Shock and Acute Cervical Spinal Cord Syndrome

The acute phase of spinal cord injury is characterized by the syndrome of so-called spinal shock, which consists of loss of motor, sensory and reflex function below the level of spinal cord injury. It is associated with flaccidity of the trunk and limb muscles. Spinal shock is not a pathoanatomic but a physiologic diagnosis.

Following resolution of the spinal shock, restitution of spinal function can occur hours or days after the injury.

A different functional syndrome is referred to as neurogenic shock or acute cervical spinal cord syndrome. This occurs after injury to the cervical and the upper thoracic spinal cord and the brain-stem. The underlying mechanism relates to disruption of regulatory autonomic impulses from the upper autonomic centers. The clinical picture consists of a loss of sympathetic outflow at the cervical or upper thoracic level. Bradycardia, hypotension and hypothermia may be life-threatening in the acutely injured patient as the entire sympathetic nervous system is separated from its superior regulatory centers. Respiratory disturbances may occur due to failure of respiratory muscle activity and swelling of the nasal mucosa. Horner's syndrome may be present. Loss of peristalsis may lead to bowel paralysis. Loss of vasomotor activity entails dilatation of the splanchnic vessels and worsens arterial hypotension. Disorientation or coma indicate involvement of the brain-stem in the acute cervical spinal cord syndrome [101].

In lesions of the upper motor neuron the resolution of the spinal or neurogenic shock is heralded by the return of deep tendon reflexes and autonomic functions. Until that time, shock is deceptive and conceals or simulates anatomic progression of the deficit. This makes clinical differentiation between complete and incomplete spinal cord injury impossible [101].

II. Complete Spinal Cord Injury

Complete spinal cord injury means a complete loss of all motor power, sensation and reflexes in those areas of the extremities and trunk that are mediated by spinal nerves originating at or below the level of the injured cord. After resolution of the spinal shock, the flaccid paralysis becomes spastic if the level of injury was above the level of the conus medullaris. When the lesion is at or below the conus, the paralysis remains flaccid. This is also true in cases with myelomalacia in the part of the cord which is distal to the injury. Destruction of the lower motor neuron cells causes a clinical picture similar to that of a cauda equina syndrome [7].

In the early phase of a spinal cord injury a complete lesion is diagnosed too often, due to the deceptive nature of spinal and neurogenic shock. Clinical evaluation is usually unable to distinguish between cord transection, necrosis, hemorrhage or edema [24].

III. Incomplete Spinal Cord Injury

If some sensory or motor function is still intact, the lesion is called incomplete by definition. Spinal cord injuries of the incomplete variant usually present with a mixed motor and sensory deficit which reflects the location and level of the spinal cord which were predominantly affected by the injury. The symptoms may fall into one of the more classic spinal syndromes [7, 38].

The anterior spinal cord syndrome presents with a typical clinical picture: motor function and pain and temperature sensation are lost below the level of injury. The dorsal columns are spared, so the sensation of position and touch is preserved. An anterior cord syndrome is typically caused by hyperflexion with compression fractures or luxations. Ischemia is thought to play a role in the anterior cord syndrome [5].

The posterior cord syndrome, conversely, results mainly in a loss of sensory functions below the level of injury. The sensory modalities of proprioception, discrimination and vibration are largely impaired whereas the motor tracts in the anterior spinal cord remain unaffected. The posterior spinal cord syndrome has only rarely been reported after spinal trauma.

A Brown-Séquard syndrome presents with the clinical picture of a hemisection of the spinal cord. One half of the cord is damaged at a certain level while the opposite side is spared [5]. This means ipsilateral loss of the functions of touch, vibration and position sense and motor function and contralateral loss of pain and temperature sensation. Unlike the other spinal cord syndromes, which are often caused by a closed injury, the Brown-Séquard syndrome is more commonly associated with penetrating injuries (stab wounds, foreign bodies, gunshot wounds).

A central cord syndrome is commonly seen in elderly patients with severe spondylosis or in individuals with stenosis of the cervical spine [5]. Central cord syndromes rarely occur further distally in the thoracic and lumbar cord. The predisposing factors account for compression of the spinal cord in hyperextension. No fracture or dislocation is usually evident in these patients. Hyperextension may cause the hypertrophic ligaments to buckle into the spinal canal and compress the spinal cord. The lesions result from tissue disruption in the central part of the cervical spinal cord. Clinically a central cord syndrome presents as impairment of the upper rather than the lower extremities. The clinical picture comprises a motor and sensory deficit which is most pronounced in the distal upper extremity. Bowel and bladder control frequently return, as does the ability to walk. However, patients often have residual spasticity, painful paresthesias and residual motor deficits in the distal upper extremities, especially in the hands and fingers.

It has been asserted that the syndromes described above represent only a progression in the magnitude of the forces exerted, independent of the underlying mechanism [98].

An incomplete spinal injury is often superimposed by spinal shock and may only show part of the above-mentioned syndromes, incomplete spinal cord injuries may also be classified functionally according to the FRANKEL scale system (Table 5).

The severity of a spinal cord injury is determined by the anatomic level at which the injury occurs.

Quadriplegia follows an injury to the cervical region, whereas the term paraplegia refers to paralysis of the lower extremities resulting from an

Table 5. FRANKEL scale functional classification [32]

A. Complete.
No preservation of motor or sensory function.

B. Incomplete - preservation of sensation only.
Preservation of any sensation below the level of injury, except phantom sensations.

C. Incomplete - preservation of nonfunctional motor power.
Preserved motor function without useful purpose; sensory function may or may not be preserved.

D. Incomplete - preservation of functional motor power.
Preserved voluntary motor function that is functionally useful.

E. Complete recovery.
Complete return of all motor and sensory function, though abnormal reflexes may persist.

injury to the cord below the cervical region. Classification of neurologic levels may be based on anatomic tables; however, some anatomic landmarks should be remembered:

- injury to the cord above the level C4 can cause impaired respiration as the diaphragm is innervated by the phrenic nerve via the C3-C5 spinal nerves,
- the sensory level of T4 is at the nipple,
- the sensory level of T10 is at the umbilicus.

It should be noted that the level of spinal cord injury is different from the corresponding vertebral level. It is common for the area of maximum damage to be segmentally below the corresponding bony segments. This is due to the fact that cord segments are higher than skeletal segments because of the ascent of the cord relative to the spinal column during growth [40].

IV. Nerve Root Injury

Isolated nerve root lesions are uncommon [5]. Radicular deficits can be the result of hematoma, vertebral dislocation or impingement on the intervertebral foramen by bony fragments. Traction on the plexuses and spinal nerves can lead to transient paresis. Traumatic avulsion of the brachial plexus usually involves the nerve roots C5-T1 with a complete loss of sensory and motor function of the involved spinal nerve roots. Avulsion of the lumbar plexus is very rare.

V. Late Sequelae of Spinal Cord Injury

Neurologic deficits in spinal trauma can occur due to immediate physical alteration of the structures of the cord. Often, however, the spinal cord remains intact but undergoes a delayed autodestructive process that was initiated by the injury. A late result of this process, from a clinical point of view, is posttraumatic myelopathy, an epiphenomenon presenting as delayed neurologic deterioration that can be disastrous to the already disabled patient. The recognized causes include posttraumatic syringomyelia and microcystic myelomalacia; other possible causes include arachnopathy, spinal column instability and spinal cord tethering. Posttraumatic syringomyelia presents months to years after the primary injury. Its course is characterized by pain, sensory loss and progressive weakness.

E. Advantages and Limitations of the Methods

I. Computed Tomography

1. Performing the Examination

For computed tomography, the patient is placed in the normal supine position. Special mattresses (e.g. vacuum mattresses) for the transport of the severely injured permit careful positioning on the examination table. They do not impair the quality of the image, provided they produce no artifacts or are not too wide to traverse the opening of the gantry. Metal objects like ECG electrodes, cables, zip-fasteners or blood-pressure recording apparatus can usually be so arranged as not to intrude on the region to be imaged. Whether the patient's arms can be elevated (and possibly fixed) above the head for investigation of the thoracic and lumbar spine will depend on the clinical situation.

2. Scout View

All modern CT systems permit a digital general view (topogram or scout view) in sagittal or lateral projection. This provides the anatomic and topographic orientation necessary for establishing the starting-point of the investigation and the inclination of the gantry. It is undisputed that the topogram cannot replace the conventional radiograph since the resolution capacity is too low. Hence, in the normal case plain films must precede CT and MRI.

3. Transverse Scan

The slice thickness must be chosen so that difficulties due to the partial volume effect are avoided as far as possible, while observing an acceptable duration of examination. Systems with a choice of slice-thickness (between 1 and 5 mm) are therefore appropriate. For analysis of the region between the cranio-cervical junction and the

3rd cervical vertebra we prefer a slice thickness of 2 mm. For routine studies of the other parts of the spine, slices 4 or 5 mm thick are usually adequate.

It is sensible to make some further slices above and below the injured segment so that normally 3 to 4 segments can be demonstrated in continuous slice sequence. So as to allow for computed reconstructions, the image coordinates, magnification scale and tilt of the gantry must not be altered. The magnification scale for the image sector should use approximately the size of the image screen.

4. Secondary Image Reconstruction

The value of secondary image reconstructions in different planes lies especially in the improved demonstrability of some pathologic findings, an improved view that is particularly useful to clinicians who are not radiologists. But the reconstructed image cannot contain additional information as it merely shows a product of the transverse slices.

Two-dimensional reconstructions are now a part of the routine program. The computed images are about equivalent to conventional tomograms, but are free from any superimpositions. The resolution does not attain the quality of the original transverse sections.

5. Further Diagnostic Measures

In patients with multiple injuries and primary loss of consciousness the skull as well as the whole spine must be examined. Depending on the clinical situation, scans of the chest and abdomen are also important. Information about a pneumothorax or a large intra-abdominal hemorrhage may be obtained from a few orientating sections. However, such thick slices do not suffice for the special diagnostics of the spinal column as its components are too finely structured as to allow an analysis of the smaller elements. Conversely, the imaging scale of purely spinal views is too small to supply answers to other problems. All this underlines the importance of a careful clinical examination, of conventional radiographs and ultrasonography as usual in the severely injured.

6. Limitations of CT Diagnosis

a) The Diagnostic Gap

The greatest risk of misdiagnosis in computed tomography of a spinal injury is the overlooked fracture. A fracture will be overlooked if it is not detected on the plain film and the affected segment is not displayed by CT (see Fig. 34). It would take an excessive amount of time to depict the entire spine by thin-slice CT. Therefore it is an essential that conventional radiographs of *all* parts of the spine should be available.

b) Period of Investigation

Depending on the type of apparatus, the individual image requires a scan period of up to 10 seconds, so that CT must be reckoned as one of the time consuming techniques. Taking into account the number of slices necessary and any possible important additional examinations (skull, thorax) or secondary image reconstructions, the examination time may reach 30 to 45 minutes. In the severely injured this may constitute the upper limit. The time required for positioning and connection of resuscitation systems must also be considered. Obviously, the vital functions must be maintained and constantly monitored. Decisions about urgent care for soft part and skeletal injuries likewise influence the time available for CT studies.

c) Artifacts

The commonest artifacts are anular and streaked in shape. Ring artifacts are evidence of overstepping the tolerance of individual detector channels and are usually avoidable by regular calibration. Narrow rings around the center of rotation, which may be hypodense, are significant in diagnosis and may be misleading in certain circumstances, possibly simulating a defect. It is helpful to make a comparison with the adjacent slices, which show the same phenomenon.

Streaked artifacts arise predominantly from movement of the object during the examination and at zones of marked discontinuities of density. A patient capable of cooperation is therefore encouraged to hold his breath during the period of the scan and not to move. In intubated patients these disturbances must usually be tolerated. If the patient is not intubated and not cooperative, it must be considered whether drug sedation is necessary to carry through the diagnostic, a problem that also arises with children. But it must be remembered that sedation may make clinical assessment difficult.

Artifacts due to beam hardening arise at the border between compact bone and soft parts. They are seen particularly at the cranio-cervical junction (skull-base, dental fillings) and at the cervico-thoracic junction (shoulders). They often prevent the definitive recognition of hemorrhages of the cervical cord.

d) Resolution

The spatial resolution of computed tomography is better in the plane of the incident beam than in the y-axis. It is limited especially by the partial-volume-effect. By this is meant the integration of the attenuation of different tissues in a specified volume into an image point of mean density. This has as a consequence that fractures running parallel to the plane of section are imaged less clearly (e.g. fracture of the base of the dens). In general, however, thin slices of 1 to 2 mm will not contain a fracture line that is not visible on the computed tomogram and is simultaneously of decisive clinical importance. False-negative diagnoses are conceivable in examinations with slices 4 to 10 mm thick.

The display of end plate infractions and low-grade vertebral compression is limited for the same reason.

Fracture lines running transversersly to the beam are detected by CT up from 0.8 mm in cortical and 2 mm in cancellous bone.

e) Diagnostic Limitations

If translucent lines are questionably produced by a fissure, the adjacent slices should be examined to see if they occur there also.

The venous channels and the basivertebral foramen should not be confused with a fracture or defect.

More difficult than a break in continuity due to a split or defect is the recognition of a structural compaction produced by compression, and based on the bony trabeculae being driven into one another. The fracture is manifested only as a rounded or oval zone of increased density in the spongiosa or in the form of an asymmetric defect of the end-plate (see Fig. 38c).

II. Magnetic Resonance Imaging

1. Performing the Examination

As in CT, the patient is positioned on the cradle in supine position, which allows for as safe and convenient an examination as possible. Prior to entering the examination room, all ferromagnetic objects must be taken from the patient to avoid injury by movement or heating of these items in the strong magnetic field.

Acutely injured patients are not good candidates for MRI as life-support systems are not conveniently transported into the magnetic field. Pacemakers are a contraindication as are ferromagnetic implants that are large or at a critical location (such as aneurysmal clips or intraorbital foreign bodies).

If uncertainty exists about the presence of metal, plain film radiography is necessary for screening purposes.

The status of the patient permitting, a surface coil is placed under his back or neck prior to imaging. This is essential for MR examination of the spine. A surface coil substantially increases the signal-to-noise ratio. The sensitive volume of the coil has to be matched to the region of interest in the patient. This allows a reduction of measurements necessary to obtain satisfactory images, the examination time thus becoming shorter. The selected field of view has to be approximately equivalent to the sensitive volume. This optimizes spatial resolution and avoids wrap-around artifacts.

2. Pulse Sequence Considerations

Spin echo (SE) imaging with its high tissue contrast capability is the modality most often used in MRI of the spine. Thin-section slices with a thickness of less than 5 mm are mandatory not to overlook obscure lesions. Ideally, a strictly sagittal series is obtained first so that a larger segment of the spine can be included on a single slice. Images in a second plane are necessary for complete assessment of extra-axial pathologic conditions, especially of extramedullary processes and foraminal disease [72]. In patients with radicular symptoms thin-section axial slices at the level of interest are indispensable.

The short TR/TE sequences are T1-weighted and provide excellent visualization of the spinal cord and spinal anatomy. They are suitable for imaging gross morphologic changes of the cord and extramedullary lesions.

The long TR/TE sequences are especially useful in generating images of the cerebrospinal fluid and of spinal cord changes that do not alter cord size or shape. Such imaging is very sensitive in imaging intrinsic diseases of the spinal cord such as contusion, edema and myelomalacia.

Artifacts secondary to CSF pulsation degrade long TR sequences. Therefore, the use of flow-compensating gradients or heart-rate synchronisation becomes mandatory.

Long TR/short TE sequences may be useful in assessing bony structures and hematomas. They are proton-density weighted and may be included in a conventional T2-weighted multiecho sequence.

Images obtained with small flip angles (of less than 90 degrees) and gradient refocussed signal acquisition can produce a myelographic appearance in quite a short time. This sequence can be helpful in assessing the high-intensity subarachnoid space and the contrasting low-intensity nerve roots. It suffers relatively little degradation by CSF pulsation.

3. Advantages and Limitations of MRI

MRI can demonstrate the relationship of the bony elements of the neural canal to the spinal cord and the nerve roots in any projection without having to move the patient. Recently fractured spinal elements have an increased signal intensity on the T2-weighted image. This is most probably due to hemorrhage and edema at the site of a recent vertebral body fracture. In T1-weighted images, recent vertebral body fractures have a decreased signal intensity when compared to nonfractured elements [60, 76]. The fracture line is occasionally visible as a low intensity area. Fractures and dislocations of the posterior spinal elements are less conspicuous on MRI than with radiography or CT [4].

Multiplanar imaging ability, noninvasiveness and the ability to directly visualize the spinal cord are main advantages of spinal MRI. Therefore, it can be performed as an outpatient examination, unlike CT myelography. Up to now, there are no known biologic hazards at the currently used parameters. In patients with spinal trauma, deranged relationships of vertebral bodies or disks are readily detected by multiplanar MRI. Sagittal and coronal MR sections show several spinal segments, the number depending on the coil type and field of view used. This is especially important in the acutely injured patient in whom clinical signs and symptoms are not sufficient to precisely localize the level of injury. Functional MR studies with flexion and extension views of the cervical spine show the dynamics of spinal cord compression secondary to vertebral instability.

Spatial resolution is somewhat less in MR than in CT but this is more than counterbalanced by the excellent tissue contrast.

The main disadvantages of MRI in acute spinal trauma are difficulties with life-support systems and the need for the patient to lie motionless on the examination cradle. In the multi-slice techniques that are almost exclusively performed, one movement during the data acquisition time suffices to render the whole image series unusable.

The examination time in MRI is usually comparatively long, longer than in CT. It should not exceed one hour as patients can rarely tolerate longer examination times.

Limited spatial resolution as compared to CT and the signal void in compact bone hampers the ability of MRI to detect and describe fractures. On the other hand, fractures nearly invariably betray themselves in MRI by concomitant hematoma even though the fracture-line itself may remain invisible [116].

Chapter 2 Bone Injuries

Many attempts have been made to classify the types of vertebral fracture, including the degree of severity, and to draw conclusions therefrom as to the effective force. The tendency with all authors is evident: a purely morphologic description of the fracture lines and the resultant vertebral deformation no longer suffices since the therapeutic arsenal has been expanded by operative methods of treatment. The clinician increasingly requires information as to the mechanism of origin, including the treatment and prognosis in terms of the stability. The introduction of computed tomography has markedly increased the recognition of detail and analysis has become more exact. For the first time, magnetic resonance imaging has enabled us to positively display the spinal cord and the cerebrospinal fluid.

However, it should not be forgotten that both conventional radiography as well as computed tomography and magnetic resonance imaging only display the currently valid state, which may not at all correspond to the maximum deformation of the spine and spinal cord at the time of the accident. Part of the differences in long-term results is certainly to be explained by the fact that not all damaged structures can be established radiologically.

A. The Cervical Spine

The cervical spine is the most flexible portion of the spinal column. Over a short distance rotation, flexion and extension can be performed to an extent not to be matched in any other part of the spinal column.

The head has a relatively high mass, so that in great acceleration towards the thorax large forces are exerted on the cervical spine. The stability of the cervical spine, which has to tolerate such forces, is predominantly ensured by ligaments and muscles. The resistance against shearing forces provided by the inclined position of the articular processes is entirely lacking at the 1st and 2nd cervical vertebrae.

Accordingly, the radiologic task of assessing stability after injury is predominantly effected by conventional views in different positions, particularly in sagittal flexion and extension. It is important that the patient should perform these movements actively as far as possible as pain and muscle control provide a protective mechanism which is lacking in passive movements.

CT is not adequate to display every ligament and every detail. We are rather driven to draw conclusions from a malposition or abnormal mobility. The role of CT lies particularly in the analysis of bony injuries, and there is no doubt that these are more easily detected than in plain films or conventional tomograms. The advantage to the patient is the more comfortable position. MRI essentially supplies more information about the ligamentous apparatus. The particular value of this method lies in the diagnosis of lesions of the spinal cord and intervertebral disks.

I. Dislocation and Subluxation

1. Atlanto-occipital Dislocation

This is a fatal injury which is seldom observed under clinical conditions. It is related to a shearing injury produced by a horizontally acting force, usually impinging on the dorsal aspect, and leads to ventral dislocation of the skull.

Plain Film. The malalignment between the occipital condyles and the cervical spine cannot be missed. There may also exist a distraction between the skull-base and the atlas, and the distance between atlas and the spinous process of the axis may be widened due to a rupture of the dorsal ligaments. Additional bony lesions of the upper cervical spine may also be present.

CT Scan. The articular defect at the atlanto-occipital joint is manifested by the naked facets of the occipital condyles and upper facets of the atlas. There may be one or more scans "without a spine" between the cuts of the condyles and the atlas. In this case, the dislocation in a postero-anterior direction may be noticeable only in a second view. If there is no marked distraction the occipital condyles are displayed ventral to the atlas facets (Fig. 10).

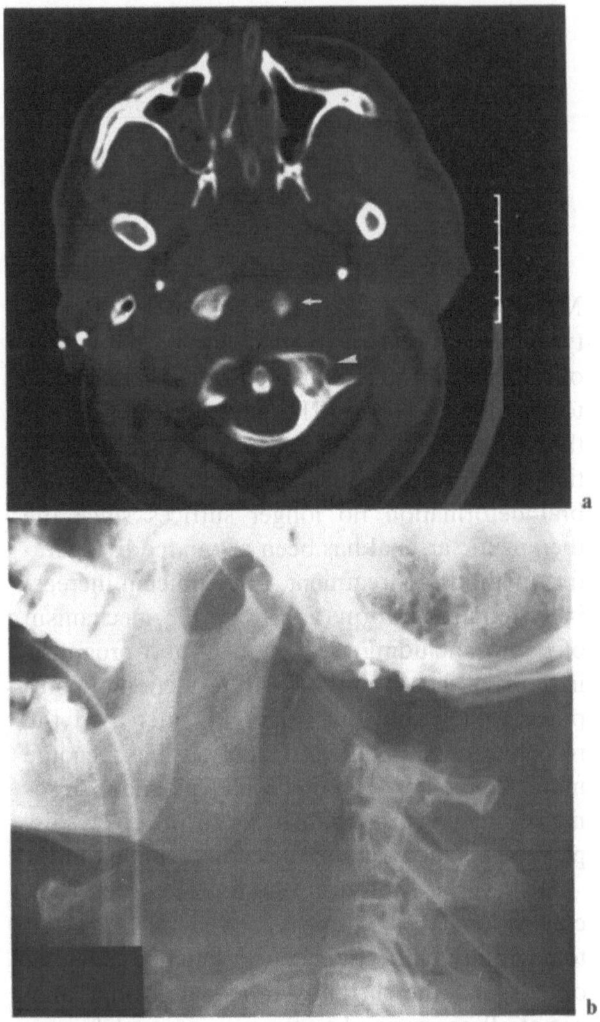

Fig. 10 a, b. Atlanto-occipital dislocation. Patient was found unconscious close to his car. Initial CT for intracranial bleeding. **a** CT of skull-base shows anterior dislocation of the occipital condyles *(arrow)* in relation to the condyles of the atlas *(arrowhead).* Note bleeding into the right maxillary sinus. **b** Lateral plain film confirms dislocation. Patient died in tabula

2. Atlanto-axial Dislocation

These lesions seldom occur in isolation, and because they are often combined with fractures of the cervical spine they are easily overlooked. The force involved is always considerable. The most important and commonest lesions are anterior atlanto-odontoid dislocation with rupture of the transverse ligament, atlanto-axial dislocation with fracture of the dens and rotation-dislocation of the atlas on the axis. Posterior atlanto-odontoid dislocation is much less common, while anterior dislocation over the dens is a rarity.

a) Anterior and Posterior Atlanto-axial Dislocation

Forcible hyperflexion is assumed to be the mechanism in anterior dislocation. In many cases the dens remains intact but the transverse ligament is ruptured, also the alar ligaments secondarily (=atlanto-odontoidal dislocation). More frequently the dens itself is avulsed and the transverse ligament remains intact, though the anterior and posterior longitudinal ligaments are also involved (=fracture of the dens with atlanto-axial dislocation). Fractures of the dens are discussed elsewhere.

Plain Film. In atlanto-odontoid dislocation the lateral view shows malalignment of the spinolaminar line and an increased distance between the odontoid process and the anterior arch of the atlas. If the dens has been broken off this interval is normal. The normal value in the neutral and flexed position is 2–3 mm in adults and 3–4 mm in children [115]. As this value is also dependent on the magnification factor of the radiographic image, Dosch chooses a more individual measurement: the atlanto-odontoid interval must always be smaller than the width of the normal prevertebral soft tissue shadow at the level of the third cervical vertebra [23].

CT Scan. CT makes it easy to detect an anterior or posterior shift between the atlas and the dens because there is no problem of superimposition, so that the relative positions of the dens and the anterior arch of the atlas can be assessed on a single slice. Normally, the odontoid process lies directly behind the anterior arch of the atlas and its posterior surface does not overlap the line connecting the medial convexities of the lateral masses. A central position in the ring of the atlas is immediately visible (see Fig. 11). Three computer reconstructions are necessary: one in the midsagittal plane to display the dens and body of the axis and one on each side of the midline to show the dislocation of the lateral atlanto-axial articulations.

The analysis is more difficult when there are other fractures present. Here it is helpful to identify the vertebrae and their fragments, searching from scan to scan to fit the appropriate pieces together as in a jigsaw puzzle (Fig. 12).

b) Rotational Atlanto-axial Dislocation

Clinically, there is a torticollis and usually no neurologic defects are present. Presumably, the lesion is produced by a forced rotation movement, leading to rupture of the joint capsules attached to the lateral masses. This lesion is not necessarily associated with a fracture. There are two types (see Fig. 13):

1. The axis of rotation passes through the odontoid. There is then a bilateral dislocation of the lateral masses of the atlas in opposite directions.
2. The axis of rotation lies in one of the atlanto-axial joints. In this case the dislocation occurs in the opposite joint and the transverse ligament is ruptured [23].

Plain Film. The plain films are difficult to interpret because of superimpositions and tomograms are often necessary.

In unilateral dislocation, a narrowing of the interval between the atlas and dens on the side of the dislocation is seen in the AP view. At the same time, however, the lateral outline of the lateral mass of the atlas is overlapped by that of the axis. Narrowing of the lateral atlanto-axial joint-spaces may constitute a third sign. In addition to these signs of rotation the atlanto-axial interval is increased in the lateral view. The sole difference in bilateral dislocations is that this interval remains normal.

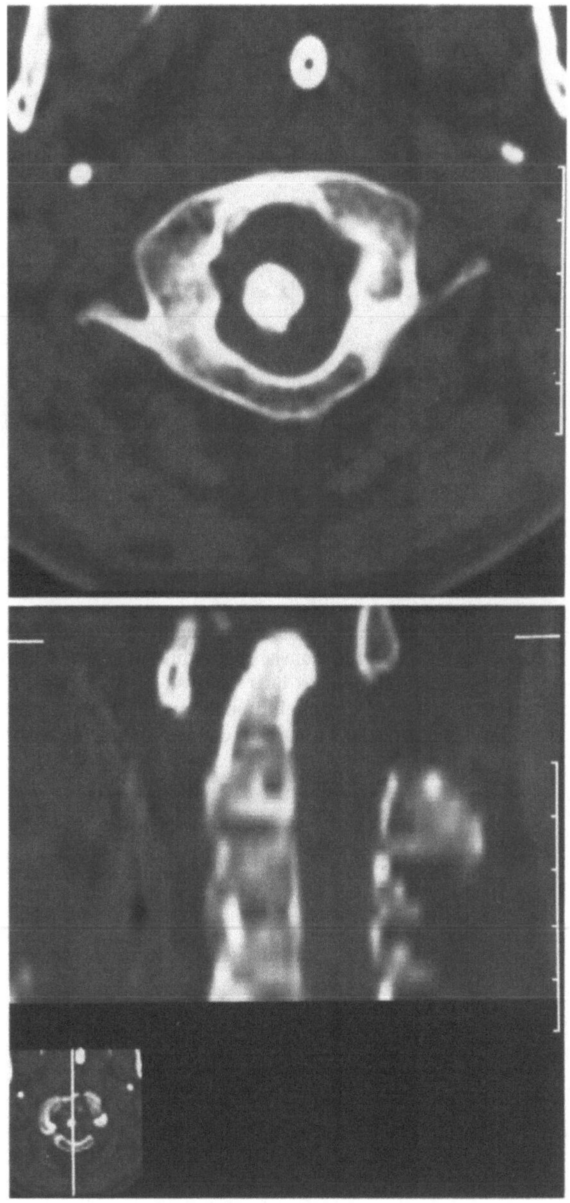

Fig. 11a, b. Anterior atlanto-odontoidal dislocation. **a** Transverse CT scan demonstrates anterior displacement of atlas ring. **b** Midsagittal reconstruction shows displacement of the atlas. The odontoid is not fractured

CT Scan. The individual vertebrae must first be clearly identified. Rotation of a vertebra (or of the skull) from the neutral position is immediately recognizable. The relative position can easily be demonstrated by computed addition of films of the atlas and axis (see Fig. 14). One can also make use of the partial volume effect in a thicker slice (8–10 mm).

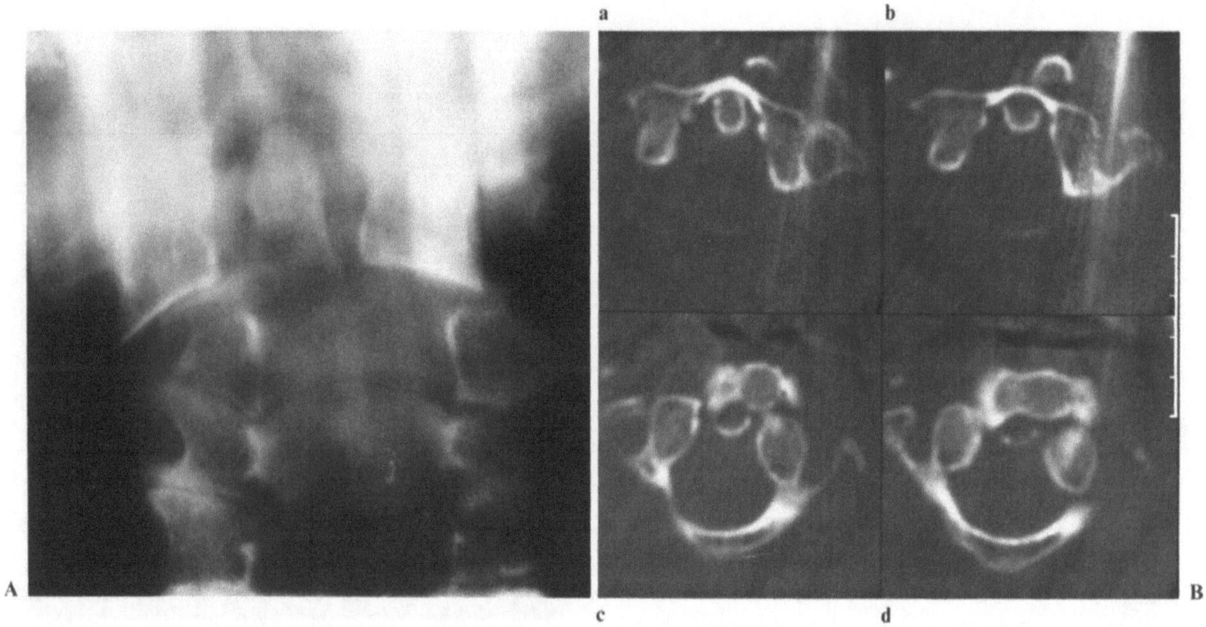

Fig. 12 A, B. Posterior atlanto-axial fracture-dislocation. An 80-year-old woman fell from a chair while asleep and came for consultation three days later because of neck pain. No neurologic deficit. **A** Frontal tomogram shows lateral dislocation of the articular facets of the axis. No fracture of the odontoid is seen. **B** Contiguous slices **(a–d)** demonstrate posterior and right lateral dislocation of the atlas on the axis **(d)**; (the stripe artifacts are from the teeth). The anterior ring of the atlas **(a, b)** has split the odontoid process, the posterior fragment lying behind it

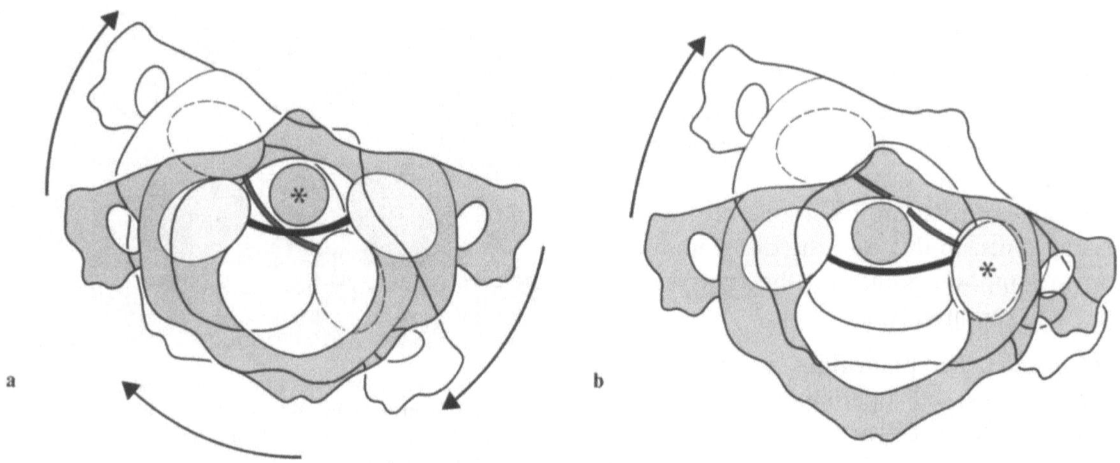

Fig. 13 a, b. Rotational atlanto-axial dislocation. **a** The rotation axis passes through the odontoid process (*). **b** The rotation axis is in a lateral position (left articular pillar) (*). From Dosch JC, *Trauma* [23]

However, it is necessary to exclude the possibility that the rotation is merely a natural consequence of a chance rotation of the head. The diagnosis of a dislocation or subluxation can only be made if the position is constant. Correction should be performed actively by the patient himself as far as possible. If there is loss of consciousness, it should be attempted only by the physician with light traction on the head and without force.

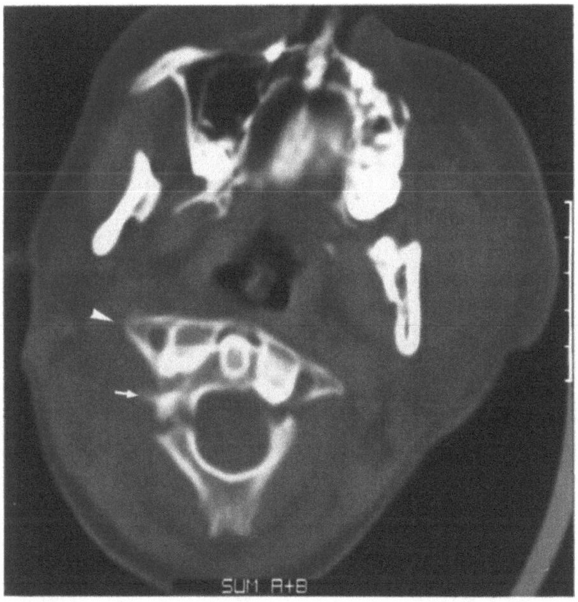

Fig. 14. Unilateral rotation-dislocation of the atlas *(arrowhead)* on the axis *(arrow)* on the right side. In addition, bilateral fracture of the arch of the axis and hematoma of the left cheek. Image represents computerized addition of two transverse cuts to demonstrate the dislocation

DVORAK and HAYEK quote as the normal values for adults a rotation of 4° between occiput and atlas, with a difference of 2° between left and right. Angles of 43° were found between atlas and axis, with a physiologic difference of 3° between left and right rotation. Rotation of over 9° at the atlanto-occipital joint and 50° at the atlanto-axial joint is to be regarded as pathologic [25].

Unilateral malposition is manifested by incongruence of the joint surfaces. In bilateral dislocation, one joint surface of the atlas lies in front of the corresponding axis facet, the other behind (see Fig. 13).

II. Fractures of the Atlas and Axis

The epidemiology of injuries of the cranio-cervical junction with the atlas and axis is incomplete. The numerical data of clinical cases are inaccurate because injuries with an immediately fatal outcome are not usually entered in the hospital records. In 38 fatalities with injuries of the cervical spine BUCHHOLZ found an atlanto-occipital dislocation in 13 cases, a fracture of the dens in 3, a fracture of the body of the axis in 2 and a fracture of the arch of the axis in 8 [8].

1. Fractures of the Atlas

GEHWEILER et al. [34] found a fracture of the atlas in 5% of 400 patients with fractures or dislocations of the cervical spine. Five types can be distinguished. The commonest are the burst fracture (Jefferson's fracture) and fractures of the posterior arch. Less common are horizontal fractures of the anterior arch, isolated fractures of the lateral mass and avulsions of the transverse processes. Neurologic deficit is uncommon but pain is often considerable.

Half of the fractures involve isolated lesions. In the other cases there exist simultaneous fractures of the odontoid or body or arch of the axis.

In the Jefferson fracture, a burst fracture of the anterior and posterior arches, the presumed mechanism is a predominantly axial compression by a blow on the vertex of the head in the extended position.

Fracture of the posterior arch probably arises from axial compression and hyperextension, so that the arch is wedged in between the occiput and the spinous process of the axis. This fracture can occur unilaterally or bilaterally. Although it usually traverses the sulcus of the vertebral artery, vascular complications are uncommon.

In the horizontal fracture of the anterior arch in its lower portion the dens presumably shears off a fragment in hyperextension. Evidence for this is the usually accompanying dens fracture. Fracture of the upper portion of the arch is mostly produced by the pull of the anterior longitudinal ligament or longus colli muscle, which is attached here.

Asymmetric compression in lateral flexion is the probable mechanism in fracture of the lateral mass of the atlas and of the transverse process.

Plain Film

a) Jefferson Fracture. The fracture is best detected in an open-mouth view, whereas the lateral view often appears normal. The lateral mass of the atlas is displaced laterally on both sides so that the space between the atlas and the dens is widened. If the sum of the bilateral offsets of the lateral masses exceeds 6–7 mm it is probable that the transverse ligament is torn, in which case unstable conditions exist [34].

b) Fracture of the Posterior Arch. In bilateral fractures the posterior fragment may be tilted cranially, as will be evident in the lateral view. Unilateral fractures are often best detected in oblique views, whereas sagittal or lateral views usually contain too much superimposition.

c) Horizontal Fracture of the Anterior Arch. This fracture is easily overlooked, probably because it is rare and the dens fracture is the focus of attention. The lateral view, or better still tomography, is the best way of showing it. A step formation is not always visible [104]. In the differential diagnosis accessory ossicles, a lesion at the skull base and superimposition effects must be excluded [34].

d) Fracture of the Lateral Mass and Transverse Process. Fracture of the lateral mass may run in a more sagittal or more frontal plane. If the course is sagittal, the open-mouth view is most suitable. The gap between atlas and dens is narrowed on the affected side while the larger part of the lateral mass is displaced laterally.

In the frontal type of fracture the lateral mass overlaps the outline of the occipital and axial joint surfaces in the AP view. Correspondingly, the atlanto-occipital and atlanto-axial joint-spaces are barely visible and the height between the occipital condyles and the axis is reduced. The medial and lateral outline of the lateral mass is deformed into a convex bulge. In the lateral view the posterior aspect of the lateral mass is either reduplicated or displaced [23].

An avulsion of the transverse process is naturally best seen in the AP view. Clyburn et al. [15] describe a bilateral fracture as a rarity.

CT Scan

a) Jefferson Fracture. As the fracture lines run perpendicular to the plane of the scan they are easily recognizable. Most fractures of this type show a symmetric position of the fissures, which usually lie directly in front of and behind the lateral mass. The cortex is sharply interrupted at the fracture margin, which is an important differen-

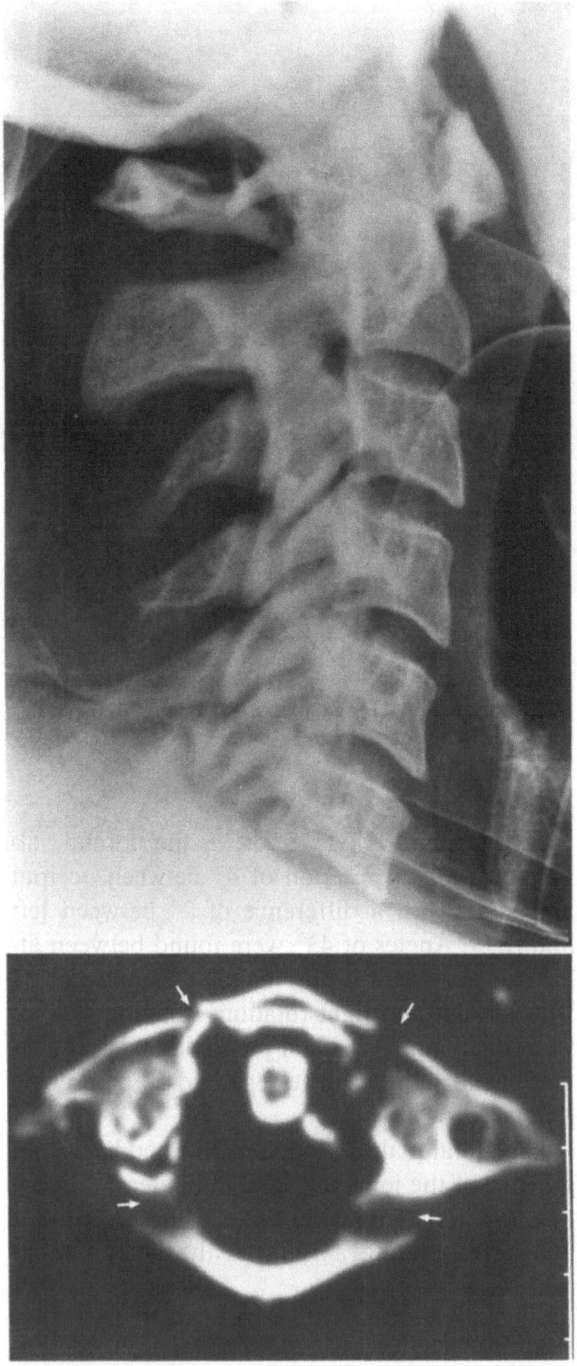

a

b

Fig. 15a, b. Jefferson fracture. **a** Primary lateral view shows fracture of the posterior arch of the atlas and widening of the anterior odonto-atlantal interspace. **b** Symmetric fracture lines of the anterior and posterior arch of the atlas *(arrows)*. In addition, small fragments between the dens and the left lateral mass give further evidence for avulsion of the transverse ligament. However, the complete tetraplegia in this patient was probably not due to this fracture. Superimposition of the shoulders on C7 required further investigation (see Fig. 37)

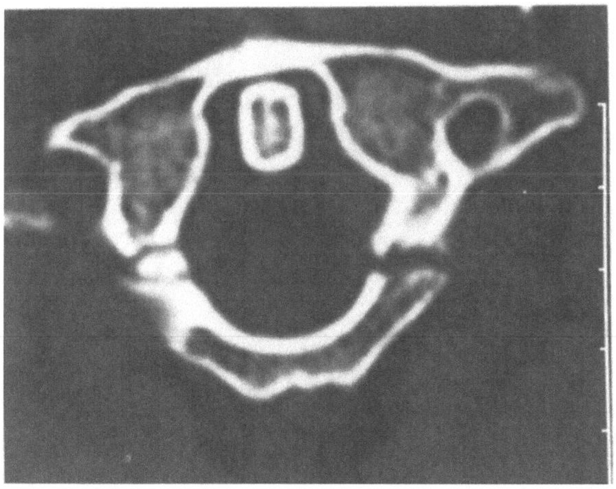

Fig. 16. Fracture of the posterior arch of the atlas. The anterior arch is intact (same patient as in Figs. 21 and 68)

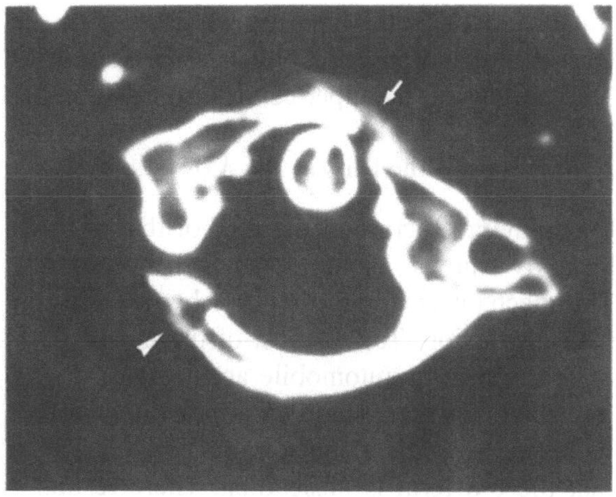

Fig. 17. Oblique fracture of the atlas: fracture of the anterior arch on the left *(arrow)* and of the posterior arch on the right *(arrowhead)* behind the sulcus for the vertebral artery

tiating feature from congenital clefts. If the sulcus for the vertebral artery is tangentially scanned by chance, the picture shows an interruption of the arch in which the "margins" appear sclerosed (see Fig. 17). In continuous scan sequence the next sections will show the continuity of the posterior arch and thus misdiagnosis will be avoided.

Small bone fragments between the lateral mass and the dens are very clearly visible (see Fig. 15). However, sometimes their origin cannot certainly be determined, because they do not fit into a particular defect in the atlas or may even be rotated. They are suggestive of an avulsion or rupture of the transverse ligament.

A deviated position of the dens in the transverse scan is suspicious of a rupture of the transverse ligament. A normal position does not exclude a fracture of the base of the dens.

The CT scans are usually better than plain films in showing the frequent presence of a rotated position of the atlas. This is always suggestive of further lesions at the cranio-cervical junction, especially a rotational dislocation.

b) Fracture of the Posterior Arch. In the typical case the fracture lines lie dorsal to the lateral masses and are easily detected (see Fig. 16). However, the fracture line may also be directed diagonally, so that a unilateral fracture of the posterior arch and a contralateral fracture of the anterior arch may coexist (Fig. 17).

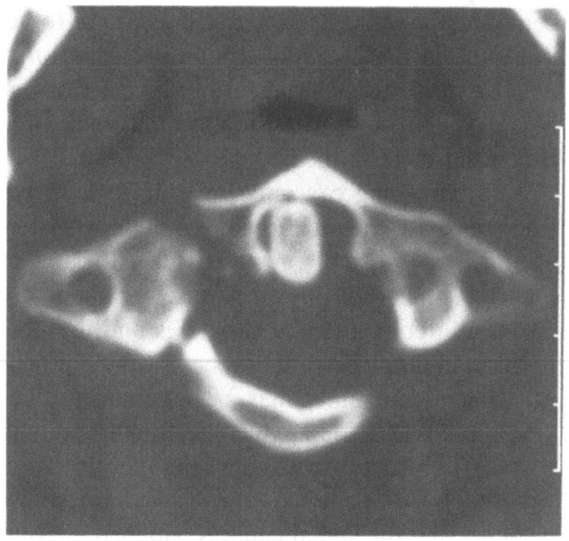

Fig. 18. Fracture of the transverse process of the atlas on right. Eccentric position of dens due to left lateral shift of main part of atlas. No left-sided fracture seen in contiguous slices

c) Horizontal Fracture of the Anterior Arch. This fracture is difficult to detect. We have seen only one case. Here there was a partial defect of the anterior cortex, but in association with a typical Jefferson fracture.

d) Fracture of the Lateral Mass and Transverse Process. Physical considerations make it improbable for a fracture of the lateral mass to be an isolated fracture, but the associated second fracture line may be so narrow as to pass undetected in the plain films. This line should be visible at CT. The fracture of the transverse process is easy to see (Fig. 18); we have noted it only in association with other lesions of the upper cervical spine.

2. Fractures of the Ring of the Axis

The bilateral fracture of the arch of the axis was formerly known as the "hangman's fracture". The mechanism adduced was a hyperextension with distraction. Today, most of these arch fractures are seen in automobile accidents or diving into shallow water. These cases must involve hyperextension with axial compression [8, 27] so that the old term is misleading. There results a fracture of the arch of the axis with or without dislocation of the body.

The particular anatomic structure of the axis certainly plays a part in the transmission of force. The superior articulations are located anteriorly, whereas the inferior facets are in a posterior position. Therefore in extension the maximal force is concentrated on the pedicles.

As a bony ring can only break if at least two fractures exist, the arch fracture is always bilateral and is also usually symmetrical. All parts of the arch, including the transverse foramen, but also the inferior articular processes and the posterior margin of the vertebral body can be affected. The fracture lines may be very narrow. EFFENDI et al. [27] found that the fracture gap in 65% of 131 fractures was less than 1 mm. As a rule the body of the axis moves forward somewhat, so that the spinal canal is widened. Stability or instability is conditioned by the ligaments.

It is unusual to find an isolated fracture of the axis, and associated lesions are common. These may consist of fractures of the dens, the arch of the atlas and the lower cervical segments, and injuries of the facial skeleton and the thoracic aorta [88].

Plain Film. Those fractures can be designated as stable in which only slight angulation or translatory deformation is recognized in the lateral film [8]. The integrity of the ligamentous apparatus must be checked by lateral views in flexion and extension, and it is important for the patient to perform these movements himself under medical supervision, with the physician exerting slight traction on the head.

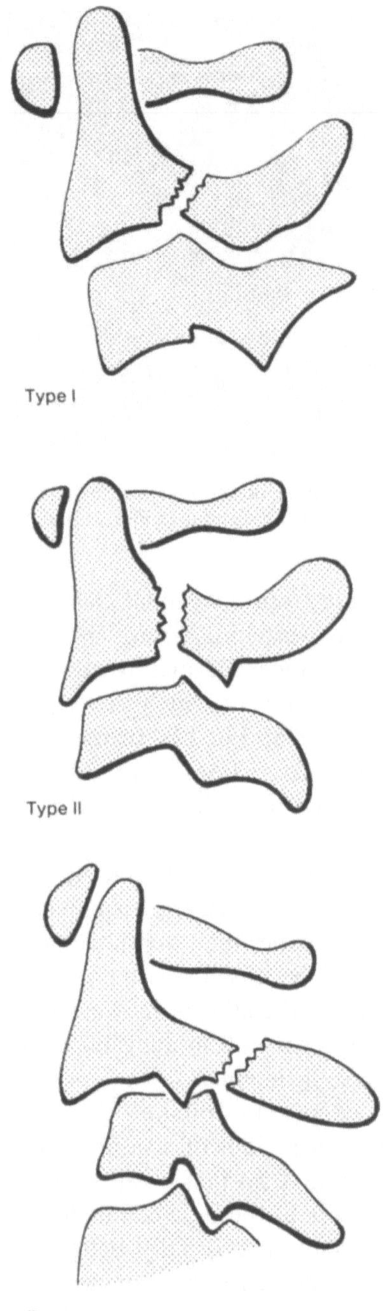

Fig. 19. Fractures of the arch of the axis, types I–III. From EFFENDI et al. [27]

EFFENDI [27] proposes a practical classification of these fractures. The main criteria are:

1. The position of the body of the axis in relation to the C3 vertebra (and thus to the disk).
2. The position of the posterior fragment, especially of the inferior facets.

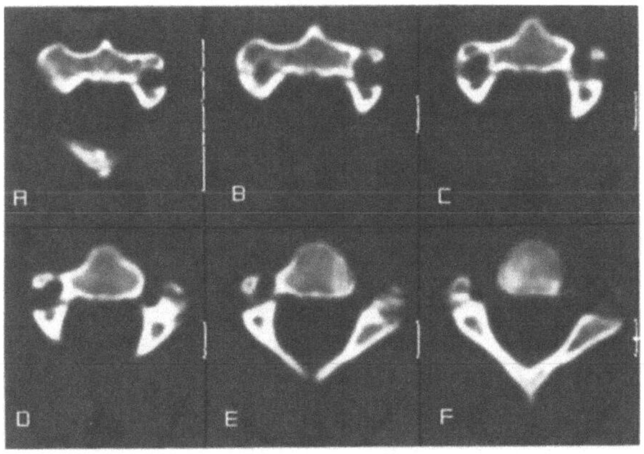

Fig. 20. Fracture of the arch of the axis, type I. A 16-year-old boy riding a racing bicycle hit a stopping bus. Contiguous slices *(A–F)* from cranially to caudally show bilateral hairline fractures not seen in the plain film

His type I consists of isolated hairline cracks with or without minimal dislocation of the body of the axis (Fig. 20).

The alignment of the anterior borders between the atlas and C3 is undisturbed. This type is stable, even if the fracture traverses the posterior border of the body of the axis.

Type II shows a ventral or dorsal tilting of the body of the axis or a forward listhesis on C3. This is possible only as the result of a disk injury at C2–3 and widening of this intervertebral space is therefore an important criterion. The lesion is unstable.

In type III there is a flexed position and a forward listhesis of the body of the axis. In addition, the inferior articular facets are locked in dislocation. This implies a tearing of the joint capsules also, so that unstable conditions exist in this type too.

White and Panjabi [115] recommend measurements of distance and angle on the lateral radiograph, which must be taken in neutral position. Unstable conditions may be assumed if displacement of the body of the axis by over 3.5 mm or a tilt of over 11° can be demonstrated.

CT Scan. As these fractures run in a predominantly vertical direction, they are eminently suited for display by CT. The purely transpedicular fracture is characterized by its symmetry, which separates the arch. Its dorsal displacement widens the spinal canal. This does not occur if the fracture runs exclusively through the posterior

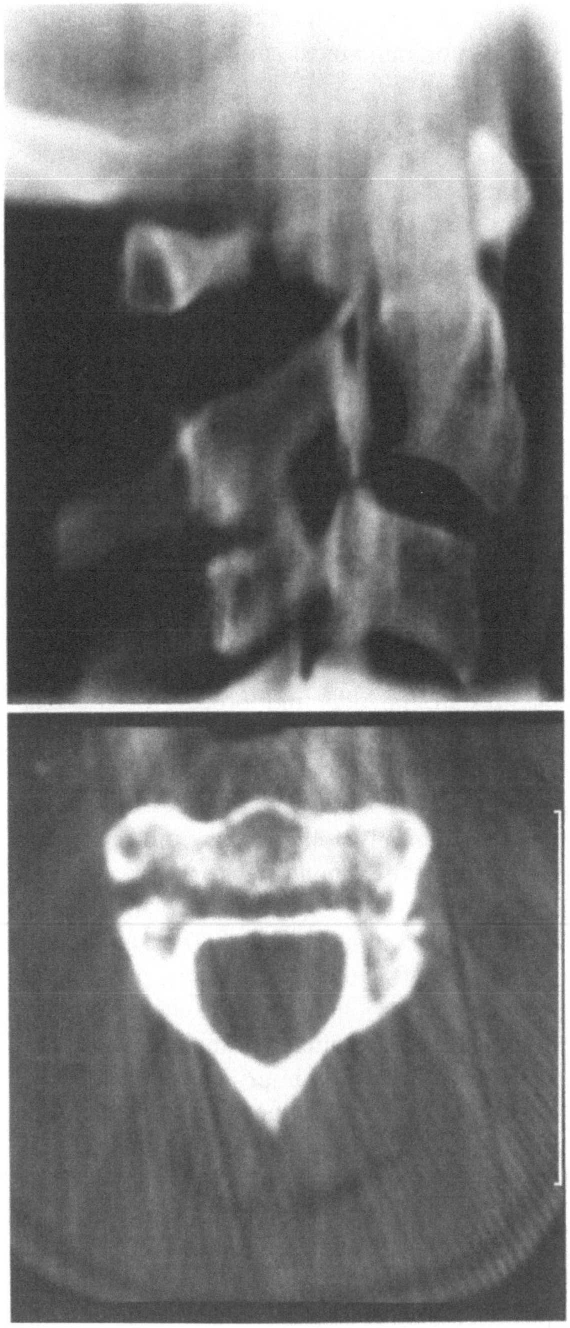
a

b

Fig. 21 a, b. Fracture of the arch of the axis, type II (same patient as in Figs. 16 and 68). **a** Lateral tomogram shows a vertical fracture of the posterior aspect of the axis and posterior arch of the atlas. Forward listhesis of body of axis **b** CT scan of the axis demonstrates participation of the ring in the vertical fracture. Stripe artifacts from the teeth

margin of the body of the axis, in which case the transverse foramina or the upper joint facets are often involved.

In many cases the course of the fracture is seen to be diagonal; it is then possible that one fracture runs through the body of the axis and one through the arch.

It seems that the least serious fractures involve only the arch of the axis. As the entire occipito-atlanto-axial complex must always be displayed, attention should be directed to possible atlanto-axial dislocation, fracture of the odontoid or dislocation of the C2-3 segment. As neurologic lesions are not often to be attributed to an arch fracture of the axis, it is essential in such cases to look for a fracture or dislocation elsewhere in the cervical spine.

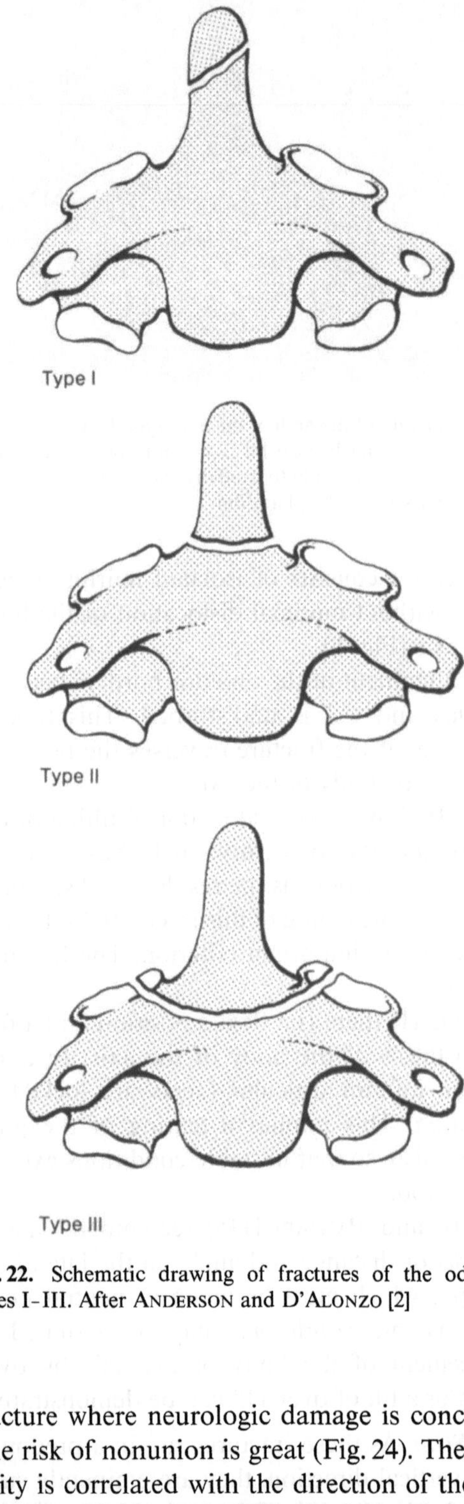

Fig. 22. Schematic drawing of fractures of the odontoid, types I–III. After ANDERSON and D'ALONZO [2]

3. Fractures of the Odontoid Process

Fractures of the odontoid process of the axis constitute some 10% of all fractures of the cervical spine. Some 70% of these result from automobile accidents and the remainder almost exclusively from falls [14]. The spectrum of injuries extends from the simple dens fracture without displacement to the dens fracture with dislocation of the atlanto-axial joints. They also occur together with fractures of the atlas, arch of the axis and upper joint facets of the axis [109]. These fractures are often overlooked in patients unconscious from head injury or intoxication.

The mechanism of the accident is taken to be extension, ventral and lateral flexion [23, 109, 115]. Experimental studies suggest that the angle of flexion and the shape of the dens influence the localization of the fracture line [102].

ANDERSON and D'ALONZO [2] distinguish three types according to the site and direction of the fracture:

Type I is a rupture of the apex. The fracture runs obliquely and constitutes an osteoligamentous tear with avulsion of the alar or apical ligaments. This is the rarest type and is considered stable.

Type II is a fracture through the neck, i.e. the junction of the odontoid process with the body of the axis. The fracture may run transversely, obliquely or frontally. This is the most dangerous fracture where neurologic damage is concerned. The risk of nonunion is great (Fig. 24). The instability is correlated with the direction of the fracture line. If this runs obliquely forward, it is unstable in forward flexion; if it is oblique backwards, there is no stability in extension. Transverse fractures may be globally unstable. In almost 70% of cases of this type there is evident angulation and a fragment displacement of 5 mm or more [14].

In type III the fracture is through the spongiosa of the body of the axis, the fracture-line often being directed obliquely forward and downward (Fig. 25). If the fragment is wedged in, it may have some degree of stability. When the fracture is transarticular, it constitutes the "English policeman's helmet fracture".

Probably because of the wide contact area and the better circulation, the chances of healing (87%) are markedly better than in the type II fracture (68%) [14].

Plain Film. The standard views in neutral position are the AP and lateral views together with the open-mouth view. Indirect evidence of a fracture is widening of the prevertebral soft tissue space, which is given as between 1 and 8 mm [87].

In type I cases, it is the fracture plane that determines which is the best view to display the lesion. If it tends more to the lateral margin, the open-mouth view is the best, whereas lateral views or tomograms favor recognition of involvement of the anterior and posterior margins.

Lateral views or tomograms are best suited to display type II fractures. Views in flexion and extension must be taken very cautiously and under medical supervision.

In type III there is only minor displacement of the fragment and the fracture is best visualized in the open-mouth view or in AP tomograms. Displaced fractures are also well shown in lateral view. According to SIGNORET [109] an additional vertical fracture is likewise associated with instability.

HARRIS et al. [41] describe an elongated ring density of the body of the axis in the lateral radiograph which indicates a lower level dens fracture.

KOCKS et al. [56] describe a possible pitfall in which a vertical fissure through the dens and body of the axis, even in the tomograms, is simulated by a congenital cleft in the anterior arch of the atlas.

CT Scan. The task of CT is not just the identification of an isolated dens fracture but the evaluation of the entire cranio-cervical junction.

The limitation of the method to transverse sections impedes the demonstration of a dens fracture at first glance and undisplaced fractures may possibly escape display. The thinnest slices available should be chosen. On the other hand, even very small bony avulsions are visible. Computer reconstructions can and often must be made in different planes and are very helpful in recognizing complex lesions. Our own experience has taught us that an isolated dens fracture is rather the exception (see Figs. 26, 27).

The first step in interpretation is the anatomic allocation of the various structures. A simple but effective expedient is to start from a definitely identifiable bony structure and to place the finger or a pointer on the same spot from image to image. This is the best way of detecting fragment displacement, establishing the oblique course of a fracture and ascertaining the best reference section for computer reconstruction.

The detection of a fracture-line 1 mm wide is simple if the fracture is perpendicular to the plane of scan.

A fracture in the transverse plane is revealed by the "missing dens" in one or more sections if

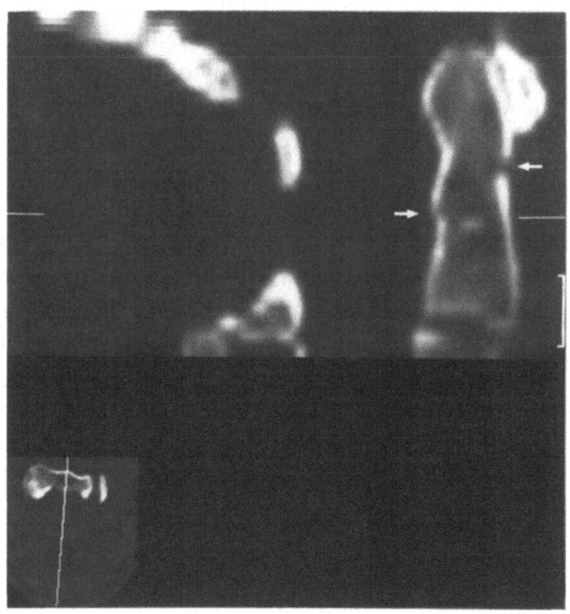

Fig. 23. Fracture of the odontoid, type II. Midsagittal reconstruction only shows small defects in the cortical bone *(arrows)*. The fracture was not visible on transverse scan because of partial volume effect. *Scale* = 1 cm

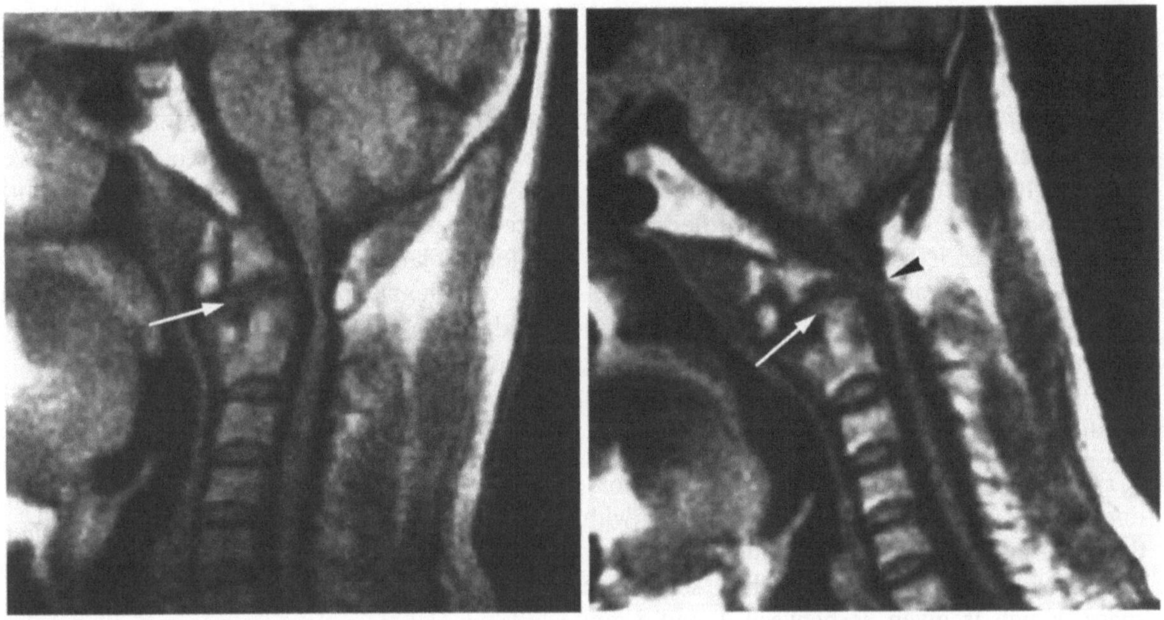

Fig. 24a, b. Functional MRI study (T1-weighted) in a patient with nonunion of a fracture of the odontoid, type II *(arrows)*. **a** Neutral position shows impingement of bony structures on the spinal cord. **b** Increased narrowing *(arrowhead)* in anteflexion

longitudinal distraction exists. The reconstructed image is unequivocal. When the fracture gap is minimal and runs horizontally, all that is seen is a dark zone in the spongiosa, usually at the base of the odontoid or in the body of the axis, which may be initially regarded as an osteoporosis.

Tilting of the fractured portion of the odontoid is most easily visualized in the reconstructions.

Sometimes very small fragments are found at the level of the tip of the dens and the lateral mass of the atlas without evidence of the exact source in a corresponding defect. These may constitute avulsions of bone by the ligaments. It is conceivable that such fragments may hinder rotation.

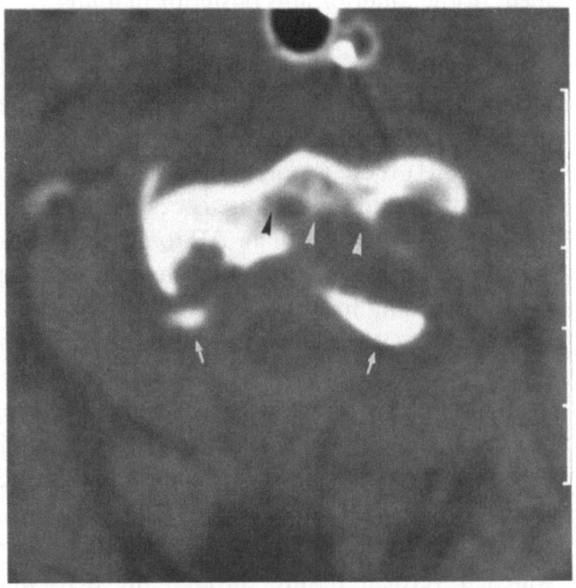

Fig. 25. Fracture of the odontoid, type III. Transverse scan demonstrates the disadvantage of tangential cut through the fracture-line, which seems to be incomplete *(arrowheads)*. Parts of the arch are seen posteriorly *(arrows)*

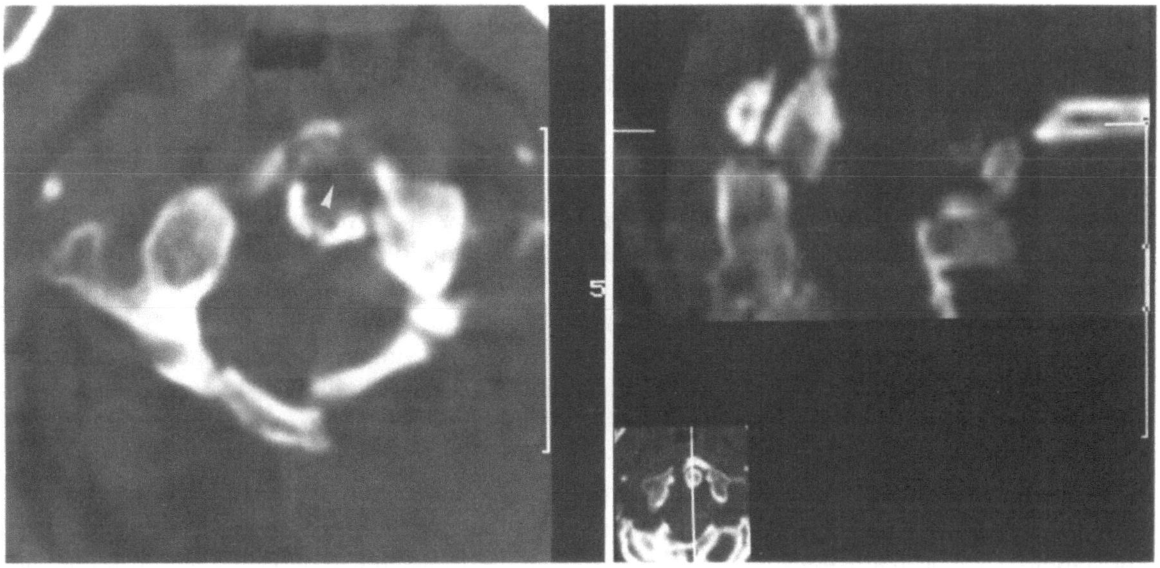

Fig. 26 a, b. Comminuted fracture of the atlas with shear fracture of the odontoid. **a** Transverse scan at the level of the ring of the atlas demonstrates at least two fractures of the anterior arch and three fractures of the posterior arch of the atlas. The anterior part of the odontoid is not visible due to the fracture *(arrowhead)*. **b** A better demonstration by showing type II fracture of odontoid with backward tilt of the fragment and retrolisthesis of atlas is provided by midsagittal reconstruction

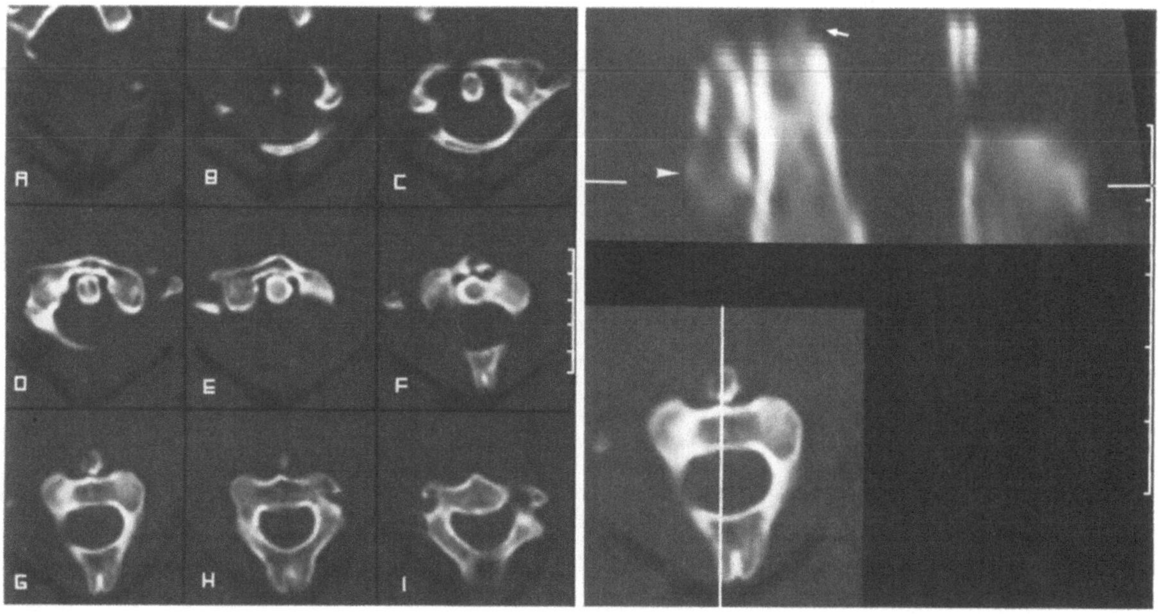

Fig. 27 a, b. Shear fracture of odontoid over atlas (same patient as in Fig. 10). **a** Series of slices in cranio-caudal direction *(A–I)*. Images in lower line show round fragment impossible to allocate anatomically. **b** Midsagittal reconstruction provides the explanation. The tip of the odontoid has been torn off *(arrow)* and displaced downward *(arrowhead)* into a position below the anterior arch of the atlas

III. The Cervical Spine C3-C7

As already stated, the spectrum of injuries of the cervical spine differs from that of other parts of the spine in being more orientated to ligamentous injuries, subluxations and dislocations. The difference in energy which leads from extreme physiologic movement to dislocation is significantly smaller. Some lesions are considered as injuries rather specific to the cervical spine and are discussed here separately [1-4].

The diagnosis of the other vertebral fractures by CT and MRI is made on the same criteria as in the thoracolumbar spine, and will not therefore be discussed here at length. Merely a few examples are shown. Classification and assessment of stability have been already gone into in Chapter 1C II pp. 25-28.

1. Whiplash Injury

We mention this only for the sake of completeness as CT and MRI contribute nothing essential to its diagnosis.

It is a loosely defined entity characterized by a wide range of symptoms, usually following forcible hyperextension of the cervical spine. Bony and ligamentous injuries and definite neurologic features are absent. It is a clinical and often forensic rather than a radiologic problem.

The radiologic clarification of the whiplash injury and its demarcation from lesions that can be objectivized are made only by means of conventional and functional radiologic diagnosis. The following signs may be observed: loss of the cervical lordosis or actual kyphosis, scoliotic curvature, narrowing or minor wedge-shaped deformity of an intervertebral disk, narrowing of one or more intervertebral foramina as evidence of a rotational malposition [115].

It is important to make a clinical and possibly radiologic survey within about a month after the injury to exclude a subacute late instability after resolution of the increased muscle tone. This is particularly indicated if there are persistent symptoms.

2. Unilateral Dislocation

This involves the dislocation of one intervertebral joint of a motion segment with moderate anterior displacement and rotation of the spine

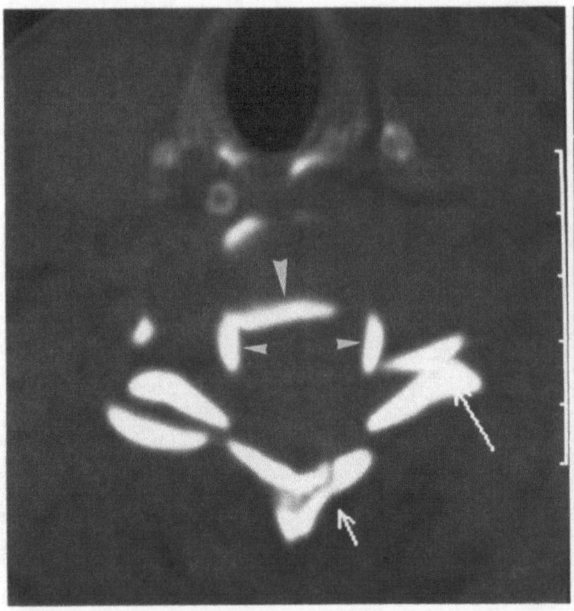

a

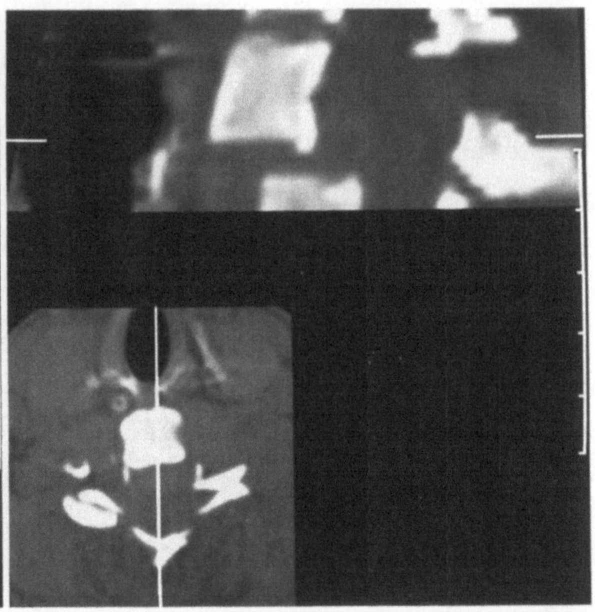

b

Fig. 28a, b. Unilateral dislocation at C4-5. Sensory and motor deficits. **a** Transverse scan at base of C4 shows a locked facet on the left. The superior articular process of C5 *(large arrow)* lies behind the inferior process of C4. Note that the convexities "kiss" each other. Infraction of the lamina and spinous process *(small arrow)*. The position of the posterior wall of the lower end-plate of C4 *(long arrowhead)* indicates forward displacement of the body and rotation to the right; the uncinate processes of C5 *(small arrowheads)* mark the original position of C4. **b** Midsagittal reconstruction image confirms anterior displacement of C4 and widening of spinal canal

above. The assumed mechanism is usually flexion combined with a rotational component. The affected joint capsule is torn, but the disk and the posterior longitudinal ligament are usually intact and the injury is therefore stable except against further rotation. Neurologically, there may be radicular damage on the affected side.

Plain Film. In the lateral view, the ventral shift amounts to no more than half the diameter of the vertebral body, often less. There is a striking apparent change from a strictly lateral view below the damaged segment to an oblique view above.

The AP view shows the rotation of the spinous process to the affected side. The dislocation is usually directly demonstrated in the semi-oblique view.

CT Scan. Unilateral dislocations are usually treated immediately after making the diagnosis, and either do not come to CT or only in the reduced state. CT is required if the bony relations are obscure, or preoperatively when closed reduction has failed.

The points to look for are the rotation and ventral shift of the upper vertebra, the unilateral naked facet and the narrowing of the intervertebral foramen (Fig. 28). Injury of the nerve-root or spinal cord can occasionally be demonstrated in myelo-CT.

3. Bilateral Dislocation

Here, both intervertebral joints are dislocated and the anterior displacement is considerably more marked than in unilateral dislocation. Spinal cord lesions often occur. Rupture of the posterior longitudinal ligament and the anulus fibrosus must be assumed. This injury must therefore be regarded as unstable to forces in any direction.

In our opinion, a pure bilateral dislocation without any fracture is very rare. We have not seen a single case at CT. It is therefore better to assume that the plain films do not show every detail.

4. Fractures of the Articular Pillar and Posterior Arch

Isolated fractures of these structures are often overlooked because they produce no or only minor interruption of alignment in the conventional radiographs.

a) Fracture of the Articular Pillar

Two types may be distinguished. The first, or fracture-separation, is probably caused by compression in hyperextension. The fracture runs at an angle transversely through the pillar and more sagittally through the arch. The second, or avulsion fracture, is caused more by distraction. The pedicle and arch are not involved and the fracture-line separates the pillar as a whole from the vertebral body.

Plain Film. Because of the rotation of the fragment in the horizontal plane, the AP view gives abnormal visualization of the joint interspace, both above and below the affected pillar. The lateral view shows a slight antelisthesis of the vertebral body. The fragment is projected on the posterior part of the vertebral body and the pedicle. Oblique views show a narrowing of the intervertebral foramen and antelisthesis on the affected side, but normal relations on the opposite side.

CT Scan. The spinal rotation may be very slight, but is nevertheless easily detectable. The patient frequently assumes a slight lateral flexion, so that the transverse slice is asymmetric. The fracture-line in the fracture-separation runs through the pillar and tangentially in the lamina; in the avulsion fracture it has a more sagittal direction (Figs. 29, 30).

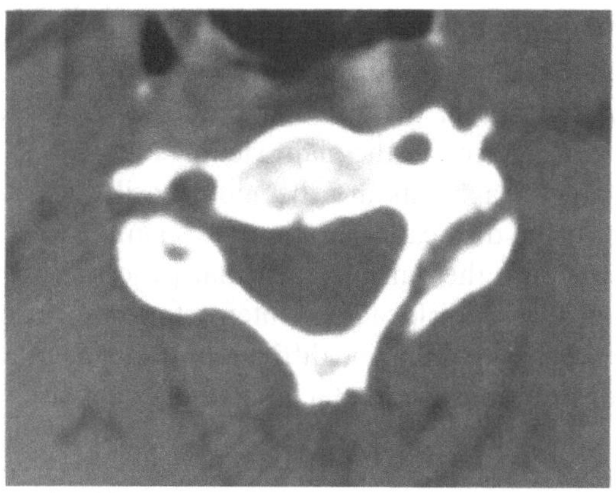

Fig. 29. Fracture-separation of the left articular pillar of C5. Part of the lamina is involved. Slight rotation to the right, asymmetry of the slice due to some lateral flexion

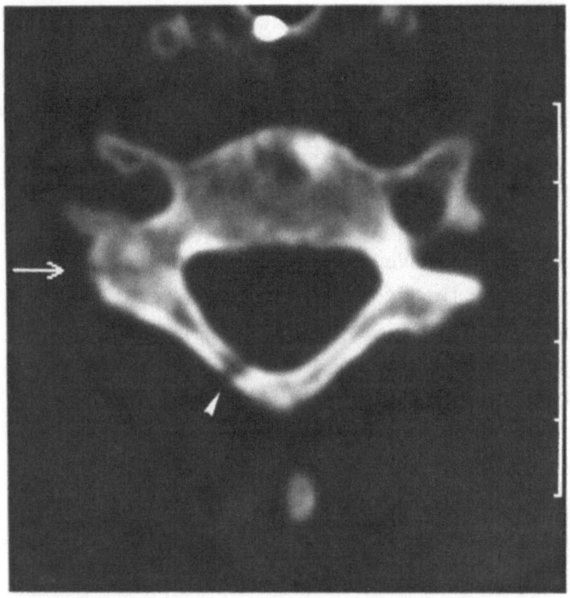

Fig. 30. Fracture of the articular pillar *(arrow)* and lamina *(arrowhead)* of C6 without dislocation. These were not visible on the plain films

b) Fracture of the Articular Process

Lateral flexion with or without rotation is considered the mechanism of injury. More marked flexion tends to produce a fracture of the upper articular process, extension a fracture of the lower. Unilateral dislocation is possible.

Plain Film. Plain films are often inadequate to make the diagnosis. Suspicious features are narrowing of an intervertebral foramen at one level and a bow-tie sign [23] or lateral antelisthesis in the lateral view. Lateral tomograms are usually necessary, as only these show the obliquely extending fractures (Figs. 31, 32).

CT Scan. It is often surprising to note several small fragments which must have originated from the tips of the articular processes as these are not detected in the plain views.

Larger fragments are the more easily visualized. If the dislocation is minor, it is simple to relate them to the damaged articular process. With more severe dislocations interpretation of the transverse slices may be difficult initially; sagittal reconstructions greatly facilitate the diagnosis.

c) Isolated Fracture of the Lamina

This seems to be a very rare fracture. We have seen it only at C3, associated with a fracture of the arch of the axis (see Fig. 33).

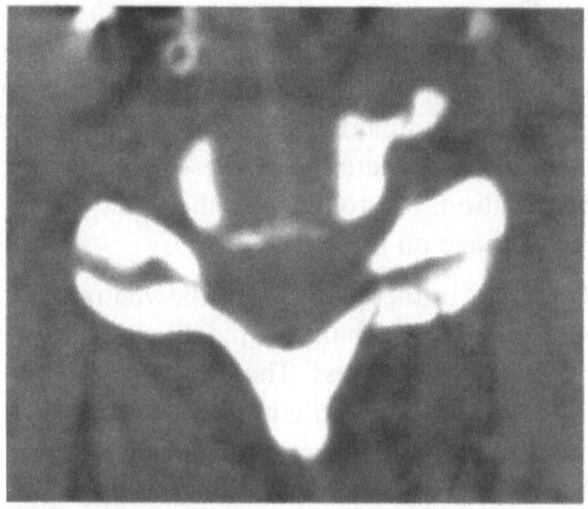

Fig. 31. Fracture of left inferior articular process of C5 Two fragments can be seen with slight rotation of the lateral fragment. Also fracture of left transverse process

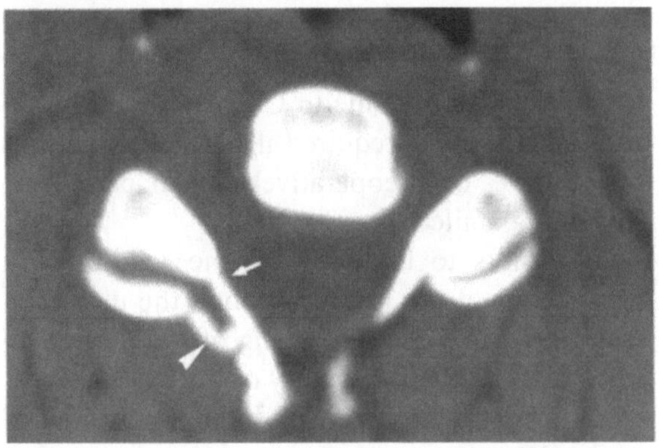

Fig. 32. Fracture of inferior articular process of C5 and superior process of C6. Hairline fracture of the superior articular process of C6 *(arrow)* continuing to a split fracture of the lamina *(arrowhead)*. Widening of articular interspace. The fracture of the inferior process is not visualized in this slice

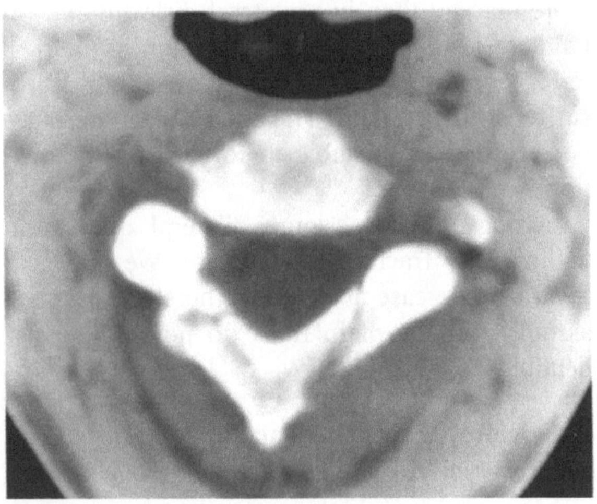

Fig. 33. Fracture of the lamina of C3 without gross dislocation. Normal size of spinal canal

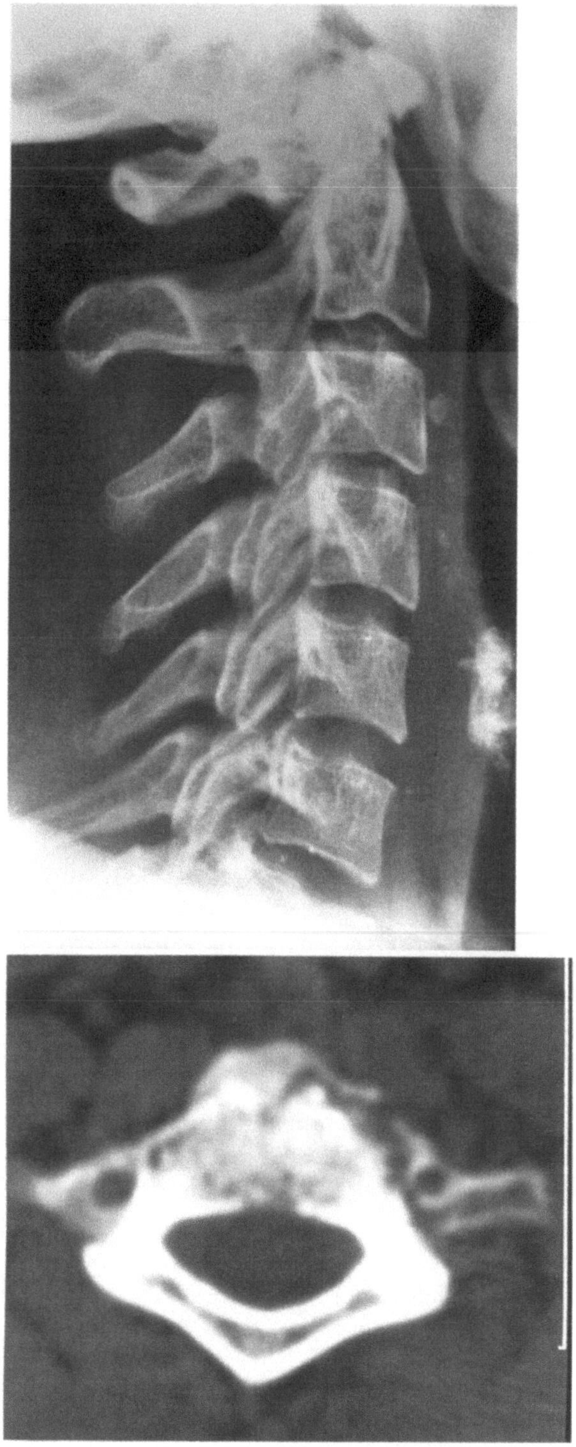

a b

Fig. 34 a, b. Fracture of the posterior arch of the atlas and stable burst fracture of C 7 after axial head-on trauma. **a** In the plain films the main attention was paid to the atlas fracture. Superimposition of C 7 by the shoulders. Minor depression of the upper end-plate passed unnoticed. **b** Transverse scan of C 7 three days later shows comminuted fracture of vertebral body and avulsion of left transverse process. The pedicles and laminae are intact, as are the margins of the spinal canal

5. Burst Fracture

In assessing the stability of burst fractures, we apply the same criteria as are valid for the thoracolumbar spine. Hence only some examples need be given (see also Figs. 28, and 34–36).

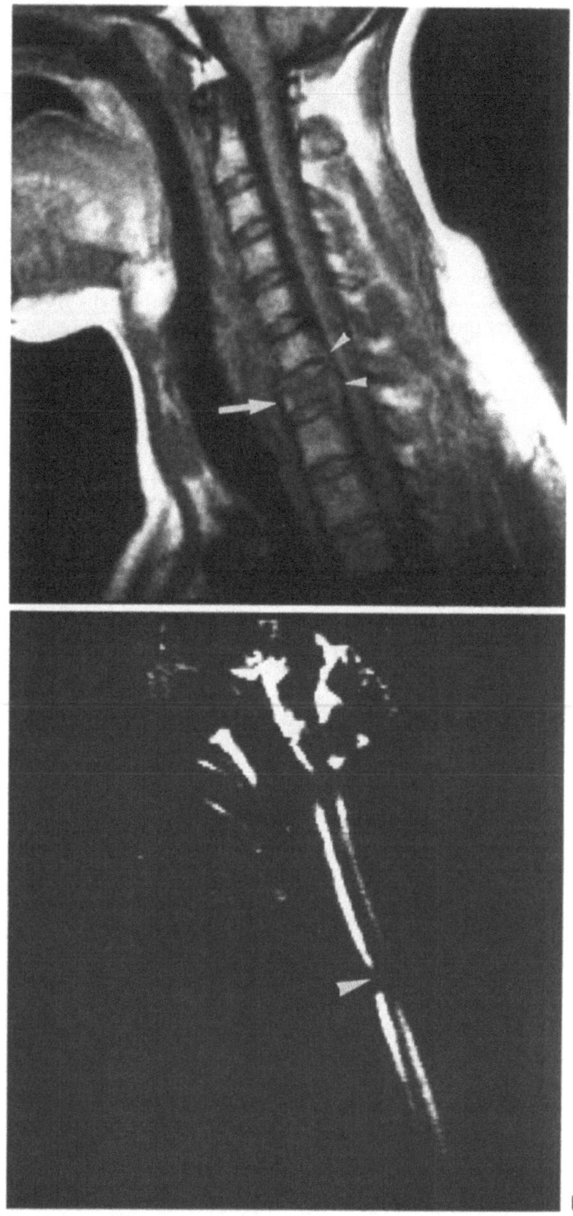

a b

Fig. 35 a, b. Stable burst fracture of C 7, MRI. **a** T1-weighted sagittal scan shows increased sagittal diameter of C 7 with low signal intensity in the vertebral body *(arrow)* due to hematoma. Narrowing of the subarachnoid space due to displaced fragment, and retrovertebral hematoma *(arrowheads)*. **b** Extremely T2-weighted image (acquisition time 5 sec.) demonstrates stenosis of subarachnoid space

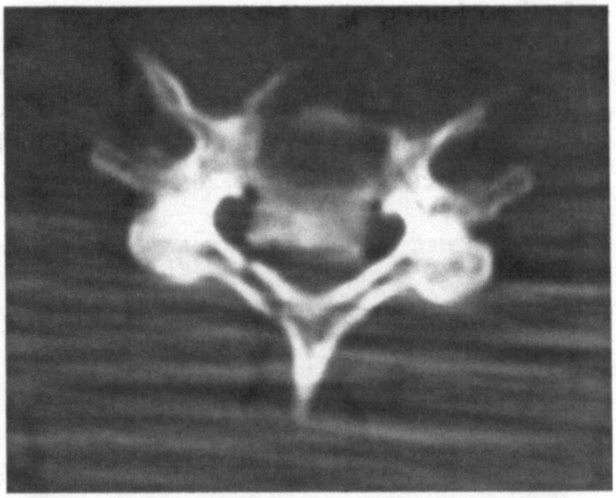

Fig. 36. Unstable burst fracture of C7 with large fragment in the spinal canal and laminar fracture on the right. Stripe artifacts produced by shoulders

6. Fracture-Dislocation

Here, too, the same principles apply as in the thoracolumbar spine. The commonest dislocation seen is postero-anterior. Antero-posterior dislocations are rarer and we have not seen lateral displacements. CT is particularly suitable for diagnosis in the C6-T1 region (Fig. 37), whereas display of the rest of the cervical spine in the plain film presents no problems. The neurologic examination serves as a further guide since virtually all fracture-dislocations are associated with considerable neurologic lesions.

In some cases, particularly in ankylosing spondylitis, the kyphosis at the cervico-thoracic junction may be so marked that it is not possible to tilt the gantry sufficiently to obtain transverse slices of the cervical spine. The examiner must be aware of this inadequacy when interpreting the images. It sometimes helps to put a pillow under the pelvis so that the head and cervical spine may lie more on a level.

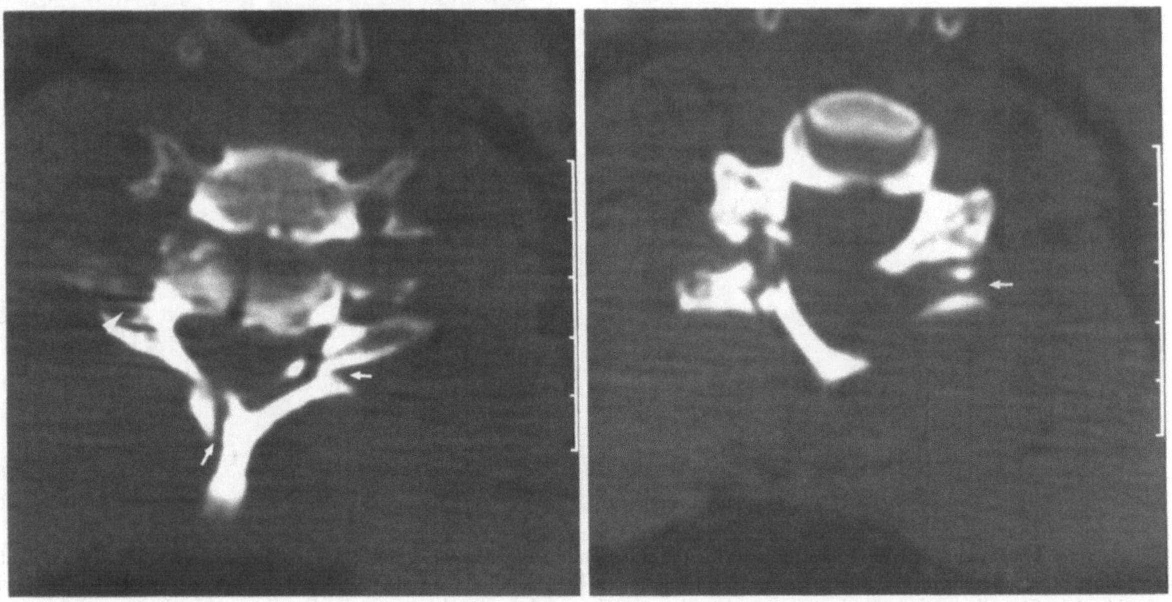

a b

Fig. 37 a, b. Fracture-dislocation at C6-7. The patient also sustained a Jefferson fracture (same patient as in Fig. 15). Complete tetraplegia after head-on car collision. **a** Transverse scan at the mid-portion of C6 shows anterior dislocation of C6; posterior position of C7 with sagittal fracture of the vertebral body; fracture of the arch *(arrows)*; fracture of the right articular pillar *(arrowhead)*. **b** Double-lumen sign seen 4 mm caudally. Parts of two different arches are shown. Dislocation of left facet joint *(arrow)*

B. The Thoracolumbar Spine

Many attempts have been made to classify these fractures, though none has been generally accepted [9, 19, 46, 66, 68, 71, 100]. The classification of DENIS and MCAFEE distinguishes six fracture types:

- wedge compression fracture,
- stable burst fracture,
- unstable burst fracture,
- distraction injury,
- flexion-distraction injury,
- fracture-dislocation.

The first five fracture types have one thing in common: they are injuries produced by flexion movement. The differences arise from the site of the axis of rotation. Anterior to this axis compression forces develop; dorsally, there is distraction. The two extremes are the impression wedge fracture with pure flexion and the distraction fracture with pure distraction.

I. Wedge Compression Fracture

The preferential location is at the thoracolumbar junction. The first lumbar vertebra is most commonly affected. The fracture is the result of compression of the anterior third or anterior half of the vertebral body, and thus of the anterior column. The posterior border with the pedicles, arch and ligamentous apparatus are intact.

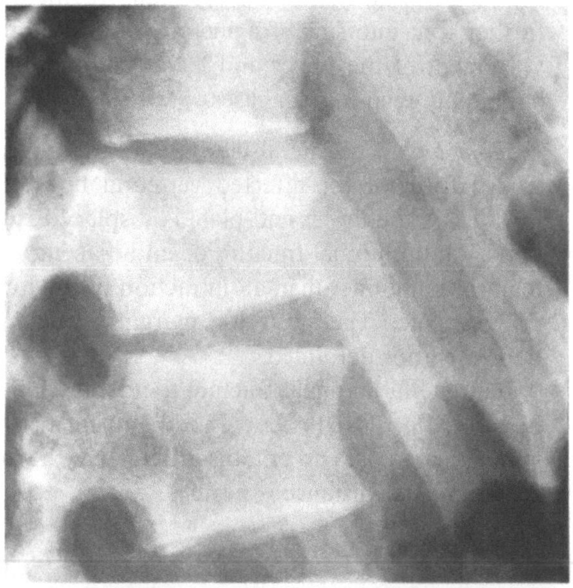

a

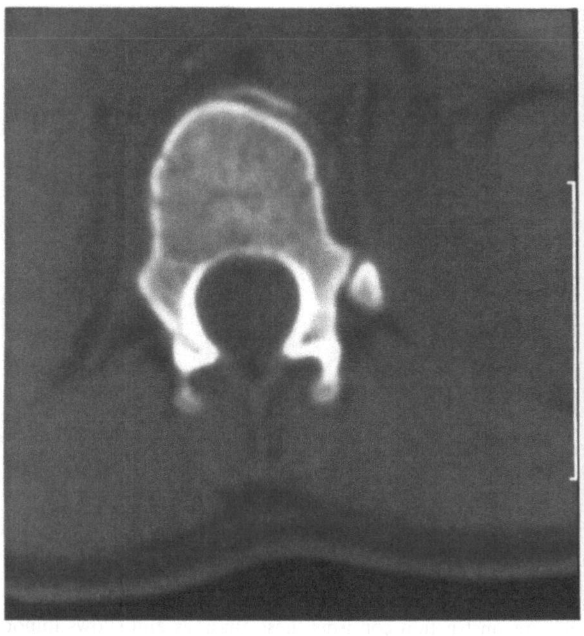

b

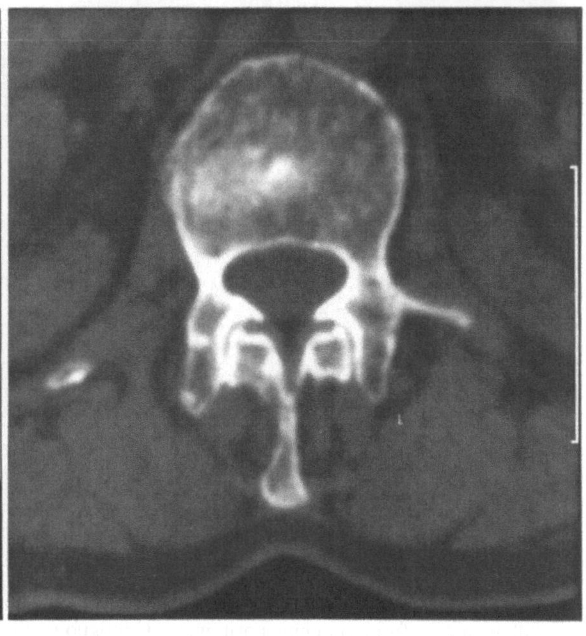

c

Fig. 38 a–c. Wedge compression fractures (different patients). **a** Plain film shows typical wedge-shaped deformity of T10, no indication for CT. **b** Displaced cortical ring anterior to body of T12. **c** Multiple fractures of anterior cortex at L1; central slight density marks compression of the spongiosa

The etiologic basis is a hyperflexion injury. Although traction forces are exerted on the posterior or even the middle column, they are not strong enough to produce a rupture.

If the compression is accompanied by lateral flexion or slight rotation, a fracture of the lateral margin of the vertebral body develops.

A further variant of the impression wedge fracture is the frontal fissured fracture. This leads to an anterior dislocation of the anterior portion of the vertebral body. Usually this main fragment is further split into small fragments. Associated involvement of the upper and lower end-plates is commonly seen in such cases.

Plain Film. The lateral view shows the typical wedge form of the affected vertebral body. In most cases the upper end-plate is displaced caudally. An additional fracture of an adjacent vertebra is commoner than an infraction of the lower end-plate. The posterior margin is neither depressed nor deformed.

In a lateral marginal fracture the depression is best seen in the AP view. The alignment of the spinous processes is not disturbed and the interpeduncular distance is normal.

The frontal fissured fracture is not visible in the AP view, but the fissure is clearly recognizable in the lateral view if there is enough displacement of the fragment.

CT Scan. Normally, there is no indication for CT. As Table 1 shows, it is rather employed to exclude a fracture, particularly at the cervico-thoracic junction, if this region cannot be assessed by plain views in the unconscious patient, and further if CT is necessary anyway to exclude an intracranial hemorrhage.

The CT scans show certain details which cannot be detected by summation in the plain film. The typical marginal bulge at the end-plate consists of a ring of fragments lying almost parallel to the anterior or lateral vertebral margin. The spongiosa is condensed by impaction of the trabeculae. The end-plate can no longer be displayed in one section (Figs. 38, 39). In its anterior and middle thirds the vertebral body, according to the position of the CT slice, is formed of markedly hypodense tissue in comparison with the spongiosa, corresponding in large part to the impacted disk (see Fig. 43 a). Because of the partial volume effect, the transition from disk to spongiosa

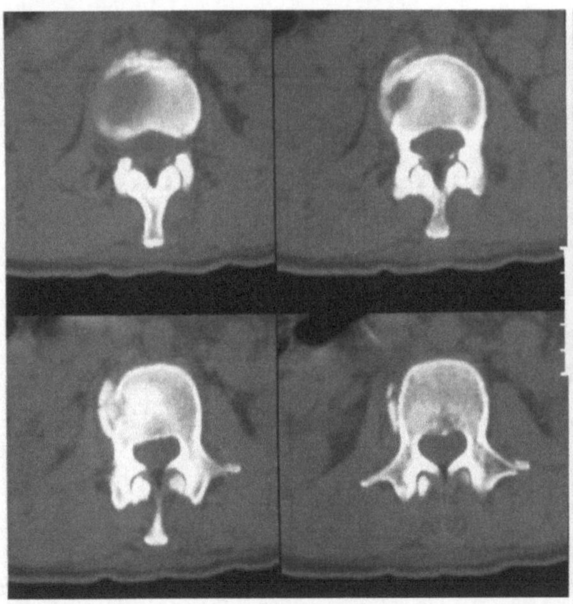
a

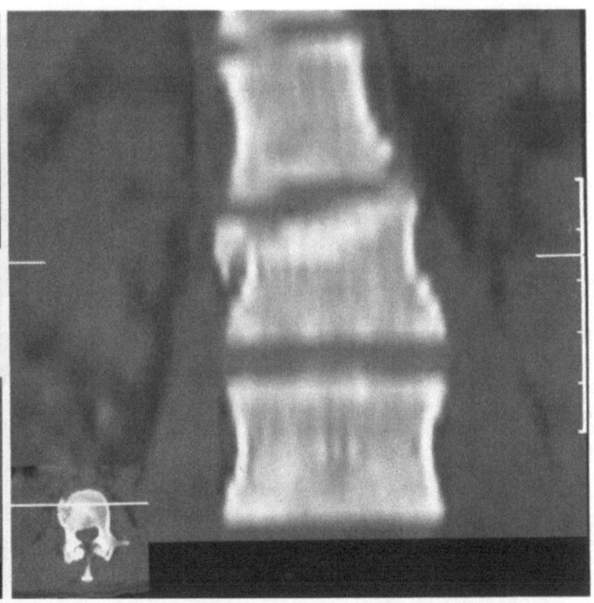
b

Fig. 39 a, b. Lateral wedge compression fracture of L1 after fall in a bus from standing position. **a** Contiguous slices show right lateral compression of upper end-plate, fragments of the lateral cortical bone, minimal protrusion of the posterior wall of the vertebral body and intact pedicles. **b** Coronal reconstruction confirms these findings and shows minor lateral bend at T12/L1

is blurred. It is important that the posterior third of the vertebral body, the pedicle and the vertebral arch are intact, so that the fracture is classified as stable.

Computerized reconstructions in sagittal and transverse directions confirm the wedge shape of the vertebral body, the normal height of the posterior border and the intact state of the spinal canal, but does not supply further information.

II. Stable Burst Fracture

In contrast to the impression wedge fracture, in the burst fracture the posterior wall is also affected, etiologic evidence of a predominantly axially acting force. The vertebra is seized between hammer and anvil. The forces acting drive the fragments radially apart. In an incomplete burst fracture, only the vertebral body is affected by the destruction; in a complete fracture the arch too is involved.

The term "stable" burst fracture may suggest that there is no particular risk of neurologic damage in this fracture. However, in view of the fact that the intact vertebral arch allows no opportunity for the spinal cord to escape compression by the posterior wall of the body, this type of fracture must be regarded as potentially dangerous. The only protection is provided by the strong posterior longitudinal ligament. This fracture does not seem suited to early axial load-bearing.

Plain Film. The reduction in height in the AP and lateral views affects all the borders of the vertebral body, though often to a variable extent. In the lateral view the spinal canal is narrowed by the broken-off fragments of the posterior wall. The sagittal diameter of the vertebral body is increased by the displacement of the anterior and posterior borders. In the AP view the transverse diameter is also increased, but no fissure formation in the arch is present and the interpeduncular distance is normal, as is the position of the facet joints. A slight flexion position in the affected segment is the rule.

CT Scan. In sections parallel to the destroyed end-plate there is a notable ring of fragments around the preserved remaining cortex. The posterior wall is also fractured, and one or more fragments are driven into the spinal canal (Figs. 40–42). The narrowing is easily measured in comparison with an intact section, but is of

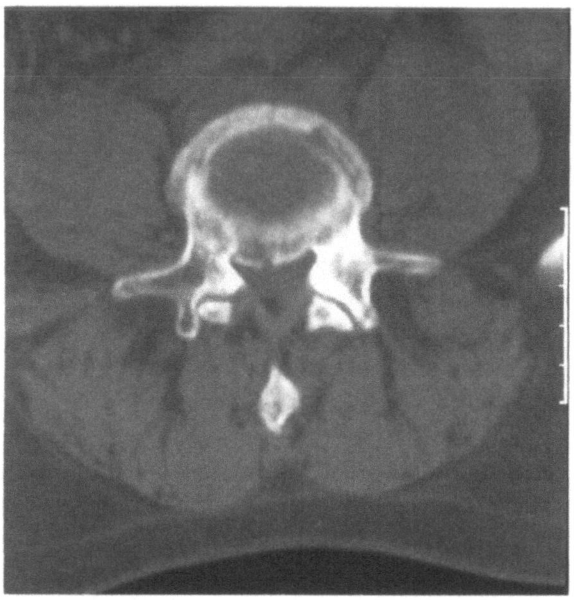

Fig. 40. Stable burst fracture of L5. Ring of cortical fragments surrounding the contour of the vertebral body. Convex bulge into the spinal canal. No pedicular fracture

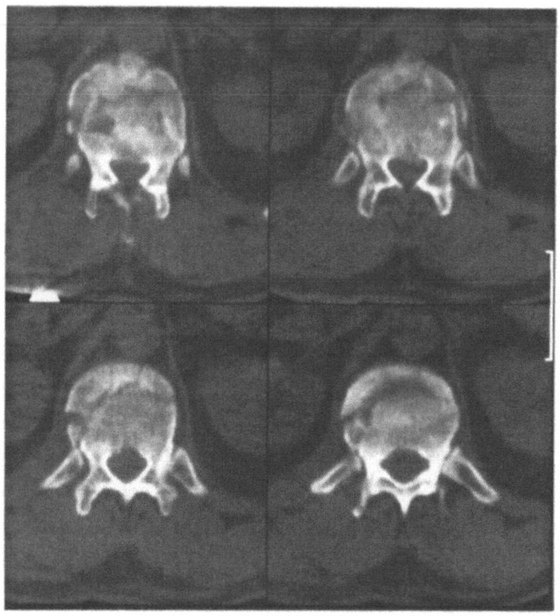

Fig. 41. Stable burst fracture of T12. A series of contiguous slices from upper left to lower right shows multiple fragments of the anterior and lateral aspects of the vertebral body, discrete narrowing of the spinal canal but integrity of the pedicles and laminae

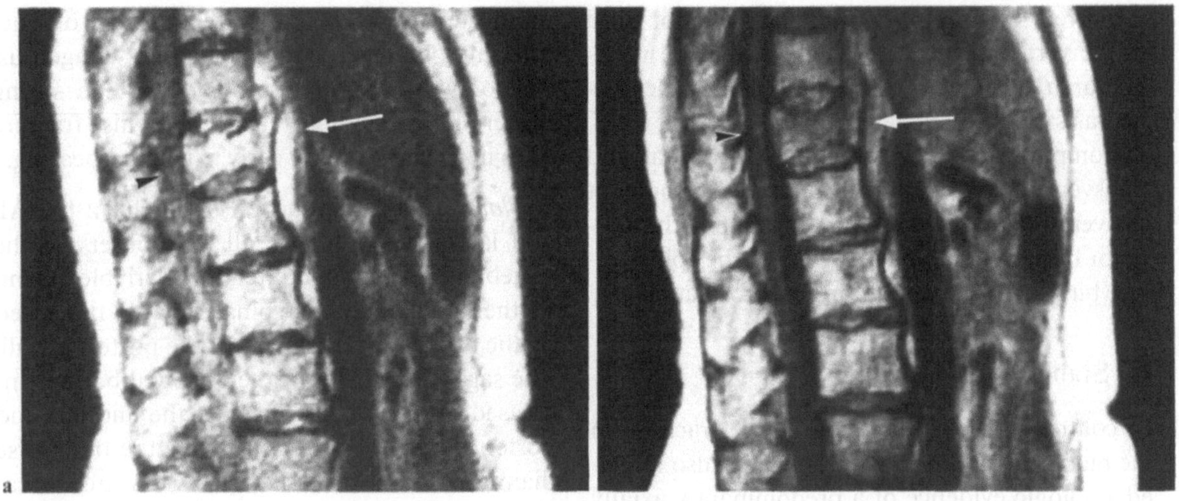

Fig. 42. Sagittal MRI of stable burst fracture of T12. Hemorrhage in the vertebral body *(arrows)* is indicated by increased signal intensity in the T2-weighted image **(a)** and decreased intensity in T1 **(b)**. Note slight narrowing of the anterior aspect of the subarachnoid space but normal signal from the cord *(arrowheads)*

relatively minor value in predicting the severity of a neurologic lesion. The pedicles, arch and articular processes are intact and the distance between the pedicles is normal.

Computerized reconstructions in the sagittal direction may clarify the findings for the less experienced. If the examination is extended to the adjacent vertebrae the reconstructions show a more or less marked kyphotic angulation. A greater degree of compression brings the risk of a progressive kyphosis with further narrowing of the spinal canal.

III. Unstable Burst Fracture

Here, too, a predominantly axial compressive force is involved. The destruction affects all three columns. The fracture is unstable to compression and rotation. The destruction of the posterior column may be produced by compression, lateral angulation or rotation. In 50% of cases there is a neurologic deficit, which may further increase as the case progresses.

Without proper treatment there is a tendency to progressive kyphosis, which affects fractures of the thoracolumbar junction and upper lumbar spine more than the segments between L3 and L5. This may be conditioned by the natural position of the different segments.

Plain Film. In the lateral view, the following features apply to the vertebral body as they do to incomplete burst fractures: the anterior and posterior walls are reduced in height and a fragment, usually derived from the upper border, is driven into the spinal canal and often tilted caudally. The articulations are splayed out.

In addition, the AP view shows an increase in the interpeduncular distance indicating a fracture of the arch. DENIS [19] states that the arch fracture often affects only the anterior cortex as a greenstick fracture, leaving the posterior cortex intact, but we have seen a complete fracture gap in all our cases.

CT Scan. The fracture of the vertebral body mainly affects the end-plates, more often the cranial plate. A sagittal fissured fracture of the base of the vertebra is commoner than an infraction of the lower end-plate. The posterior wall is split into multiple fragments and driven into the spinal canal, which is not uncommonly narrowed by more than 50%. The interpeduncular distance is enlarged, often by only a few millimeters. The cause is plainly visible: one or more fractures of the arch and loss of contact between the pedicles and the vertebral body (Figs. 43–45). Here the fracture-lines usually run obliquely. The articular processes are not necessarily broken off, but this is always the case in lumbar fractures if there is also a rotational component. This is evidenced

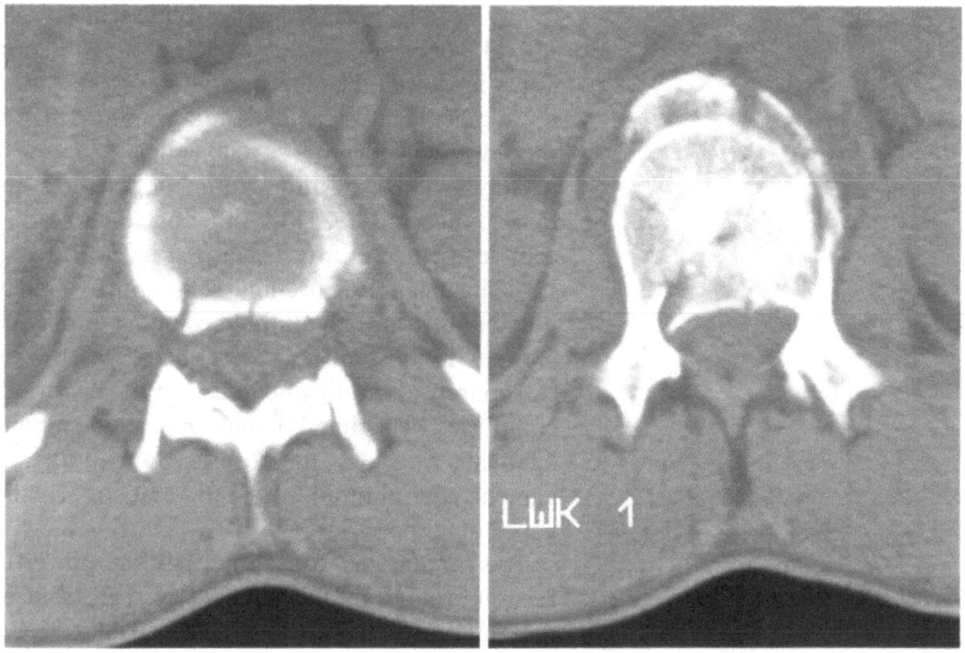

a b

Fig. 43 a, b. Unstable burst fracture of L1. **a** Slice through upper end-plate, which is fragmented. Central herniation of disk material. **b** Slice 4 mm caudally. Narrowing of spinal canal by fragment of posterior aspect of vertebral body

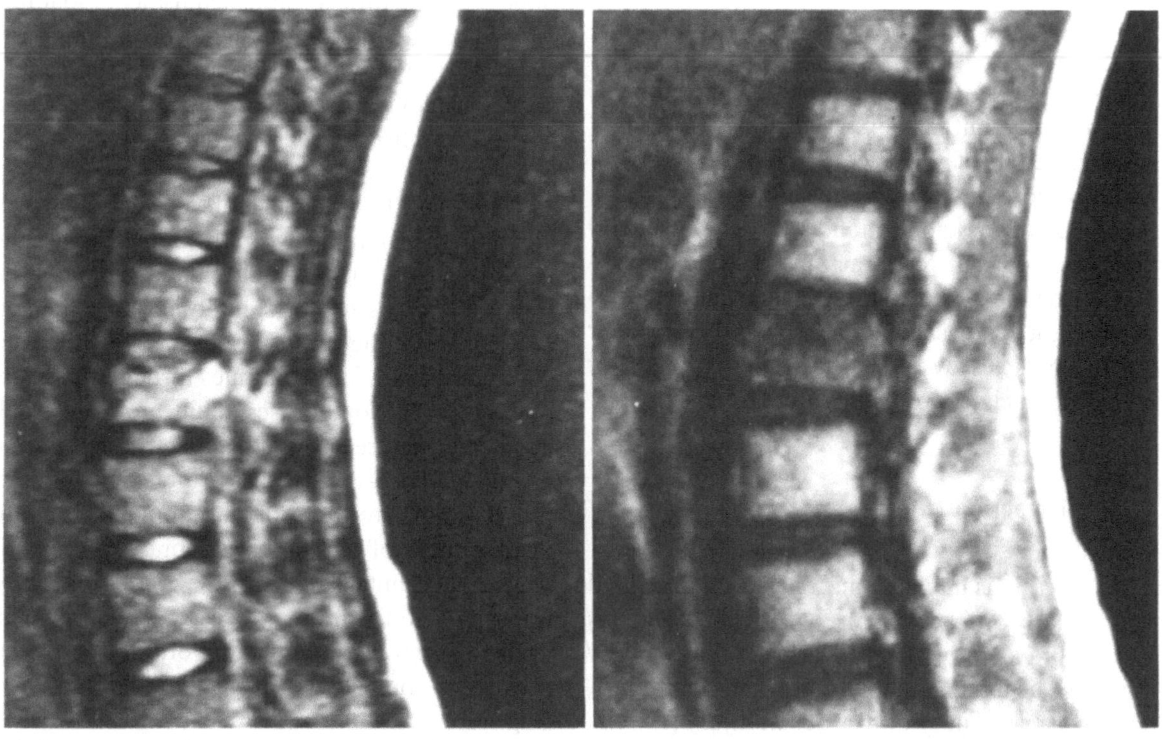

a b

Fig. 44. Unstable burst fracture of T12, sagittal MRI. **a** T2-weighted image shows increased signal intensity of the vertebral body and marked narrowing of spinal canal. **b** Decreased signal intensity in T1-weighted image

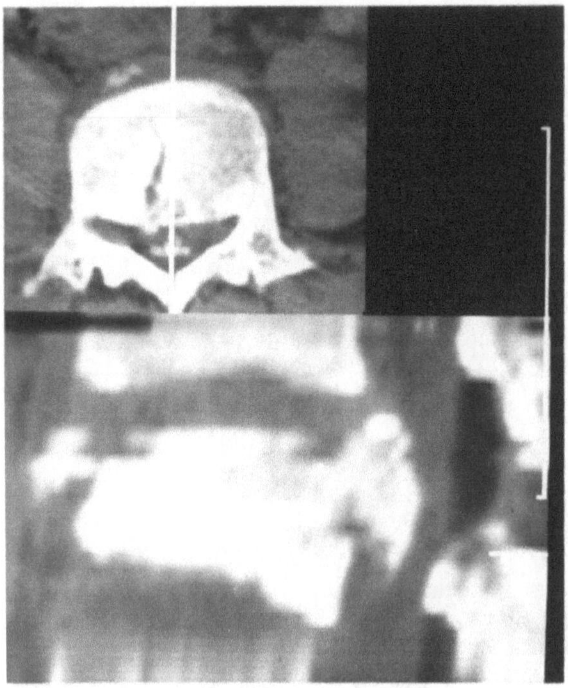

Fig. 45. Unstable burst fracture of L3. No initial neurologic deficit. Diagnosis missed on plain film. Bladder dysfunction developed 5 weeks later. Transverse CT scan and sagittal reconstruction show sagittal cleft through vertebral body and midline of arch (superimposed by reconstruction line) and marked narrowing of spinal canal

not only by the different rotational position of the vertebrae but also by the fact that the reduction in height of the fractured vertebral body is usually more marked on one side.

If operative stabilization is under consideration, the adjacent vertebrae must also be displayed to exclude a fracture. If a fixateur interne is to be used, it is advisable to determine the diameter of the pedicles by CT as these must be greater than the thickness of the intended screws.

IV. Distraction Injury

This fracture is uncommon. It has been described particularly in the victims of driving accidents who wore a simple lap-belt. This is indicated by the various terms: seat-belt injury, lap-belt injury, seat-belt type injury or distraction injury [19, 110, 113]. The incidence in our own country has at least fallen since the use of three-point belts. This fracture can be regarded as a specific type [19, 68, 110, 113] or as a special case of flexion-distraction injury in view of the mechanism. The preservation of stability against axial loading argues that it should be considered a special entity.

Only 4-5% of all thoracolumbar fractures belong to this type [19, 113]. Either one or two adjacent segments are affected at the level of T1 to L4. The main fracture-line runs approximately horizontally through all three columns. It may be entirely intraosseous as described by CHANCE [13], purely disko-ligamentous, or traverse both complexes. The interspinous and supraspinous ligaments as well as the posterior longitudinal ligaments are ruptured, so that the fracture usually gapes open posteriorly.

This implies as causal mechanism powerful flexion around an axis situated at or in front of the anterior vertebral border, the greatest physical component of the force being an axial distraction.

As all three columns are damaged, the fracture is unstable, particularly in rotation and flexion. The anterior border of the vertebra acts as a hinge around which the fracture cleft gapes open. The fracture is stable against axial loading.

Associated injuries in the form of blunt abdominal trauma are often present. These are more probably produced by force exerted in a sagittal direction.

Plain Film. The most useful information is provided by the lateral view. In the bony fracture the fracture edges open dorsally like a scissors. The fracture-line passes horizontally through the spinous process, the arch, the transverse processes and the pedicles and continues through the vertebral body. In some cases there are very small avulsion fractures from the anterior margin of the body. The articulation of the small joints is preserved. There is no or only minimal forward displacement of the upper vertebra.

The horizontal cleft in the vertebral body, transverse and spinous processes is also evident in the AP view, while breaking-off of an articular process is best detected in the oblique view (Fig. 46).

The main feature of the predominantly disko-ligamentous type is the marked increase of the

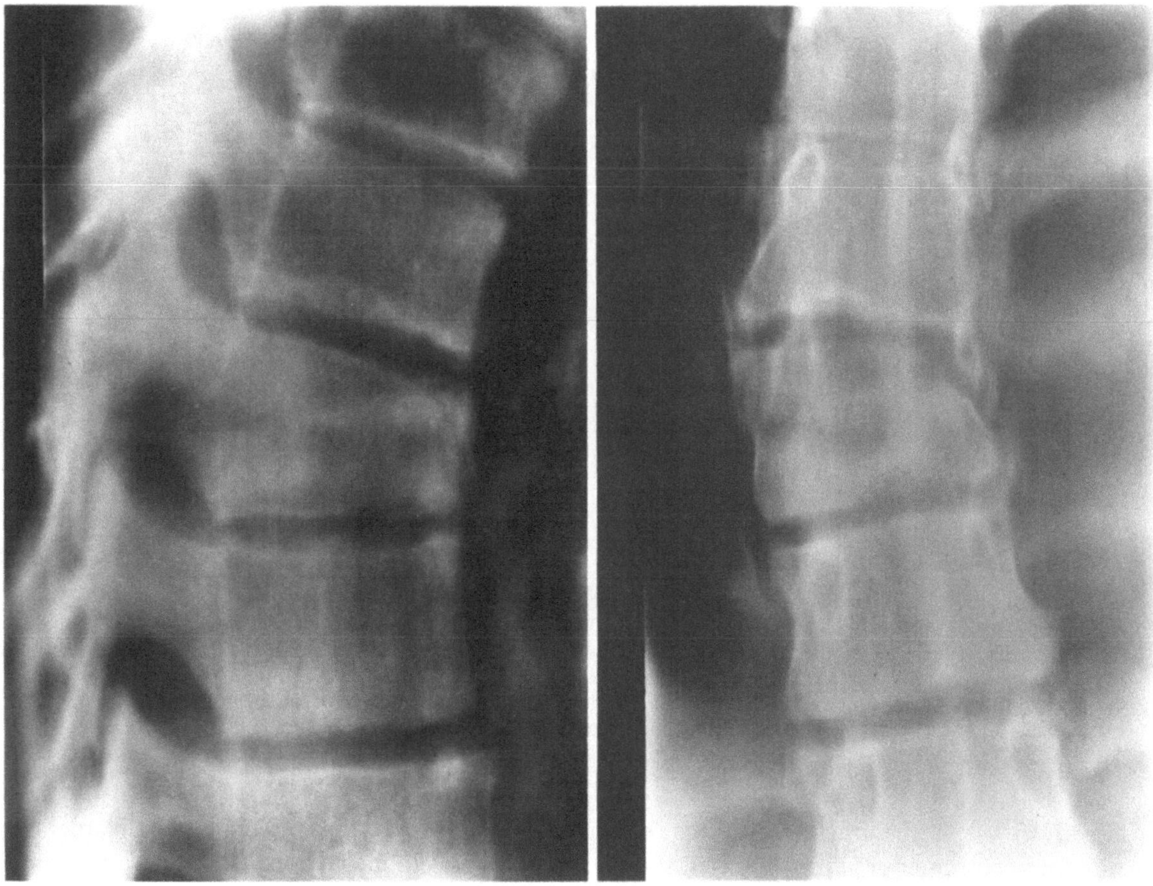

a b

Fig. 46. Distraction injury (Chance fracture) of T10. **a** Nearly horizontal fracture-line through vertebral body with dorsal gap. Widening of intervertebral foramen. No forward displacement of upper vertebra. **b** AP view shows somewhat oblique cleft in vertebral body and consequent lateral bend of vertebral column. (CT not done)

distance between the spinous processes, evidence of rupture of the supraspinous and interspinous ligaments. The facet joint spaces may be considerably widened. The disk-space is opened dorsally and of normal width ventrally. The alignment of the anterior spinal contour is not interrupted.

As this type of fracture is unstable in forward and lateral flexion and also in rotation, the AP view may also show a lateral tilt or a minor rotation above the ruptured disk, depending on the nature of the injury.

Usually the injury combines bony and diskoligamentous features; there is usually destruction of the posterior ligamentous complex from which a transpedicular fracture radiates obliquely caudally into the posterior wall of the vertebral border. Continuation into the adjacent lower disk space is evidenced by dorsal widening.

CT Scan. In the bony type, the somewhat difficult diagnosis from the CT findings depends on three factors:

1. the width of the fracture gap in the vertebral body and spinous process,
2. the slice thickness used, and
3. the direction of the fracture in relation to the scan plane.

If the fracture runs horizontally and the slice thickness is 5 mm or more the fracture may be overlooked. But the course is usually oblique and the fractures are detectable, particularly in the pars interarticularis and the posterior third of the vertebral body and in avulsion fractures of the articular processes.

Computer reconstructions based on thin slices give images that show much the same signs as

a 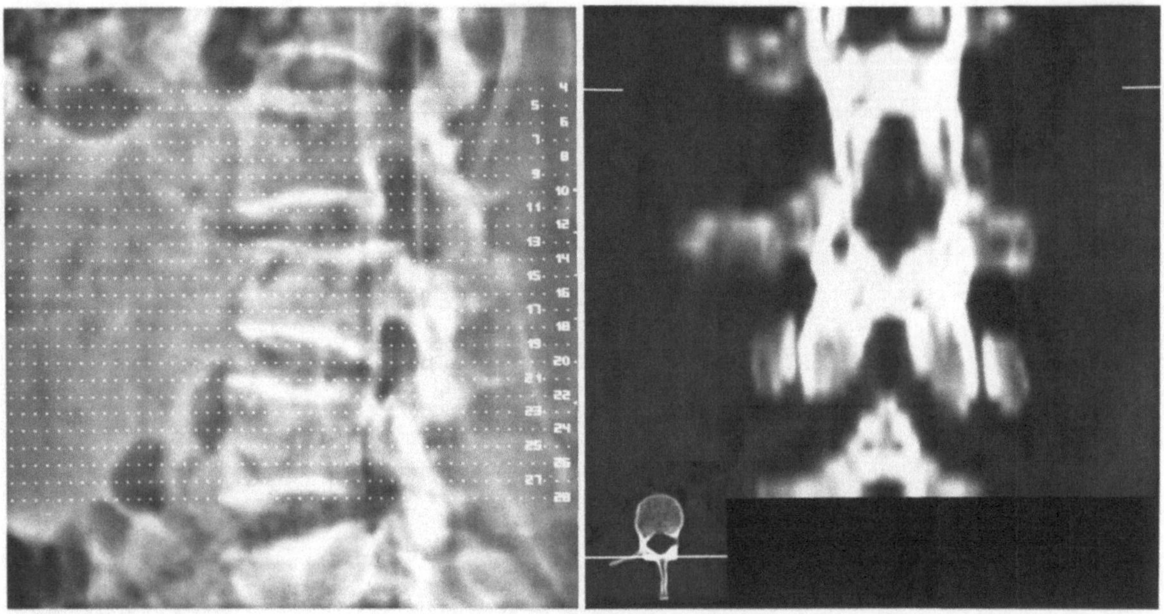 b

Fig. 47 a, b. Disko-ligamentous type of distraction injury at L1–2. **a** Lateral topogram shows minimal antelisthesis of L1 and discrete widening of the intervertebral foramen. Anterior longitudinal ligament probably intact. Contiguous slices *(line 4 to 28)* showed no bony lesion. **b** Coronal reconstruction through facet joints and articular processes demonstrates symmetric loss of articulation

lateral views. If the fracture is wedge-shaped with an open posterior gap, this is well shown as is the increased distance between the spinous processes, and display of the kyphotic angulation also depends on this.

No, or only very small, fragments are demonstrable at the anterior border.

In the disko-ligamentous type, an exposed ("naked") facet is observable in several consecutive transverse slices, indirectly implying the associated rupture of the joint capsule. The same applies to demonstration of rupture of the dorsal ligaments including the ligamenta flava (Fig. 47).

V. Flexion-Distraction Injury

Here again a hyperflexion mechanism is involved, but with the special feature that the rotation point is not situated at or in front of the anterior border of the spine but between the anterior and posterior longitudinal ligaments. Hence distraction forces are exerted on the middle and posterior columns but axial compression on the anterior column. Denis counts this as a form of fracture-dislocation. What is involved is an osteo-disko-ligamentous fracture.

The supra- and interspinous ligaments are torn, and in most cases so is the posterior longitudinal ligament, or at least overstretched. Therefore the fracture may gape dorsally. Whether there is a dislocation of the small articulations depends on the course of the fracture. If this runs through the arch and the articular processes, the articulation cranial and caudal to it may be normal. However, it often runs through the joint-space, which may be opened up by the kyphotic angulation and the posterior border of the vertebral body may remain uninjured.

At the vertebral body, the injury may produce either a comminuted fracture of the upper vertebra or of the end-plate of the lower vertebra. This is a further distinguishing feature from distraction fracture. If the posterior border is also affected there will be a fragment in the spinal canal because there is no support from the posterior longitudinal ligament. A disk rupture may occur. The fracture is unstable in flexion, distraction and in rotation.

Plain Film. In the lateral film the kyphotic angulation is evident and is associated with reduced height of the anterior border and splaying

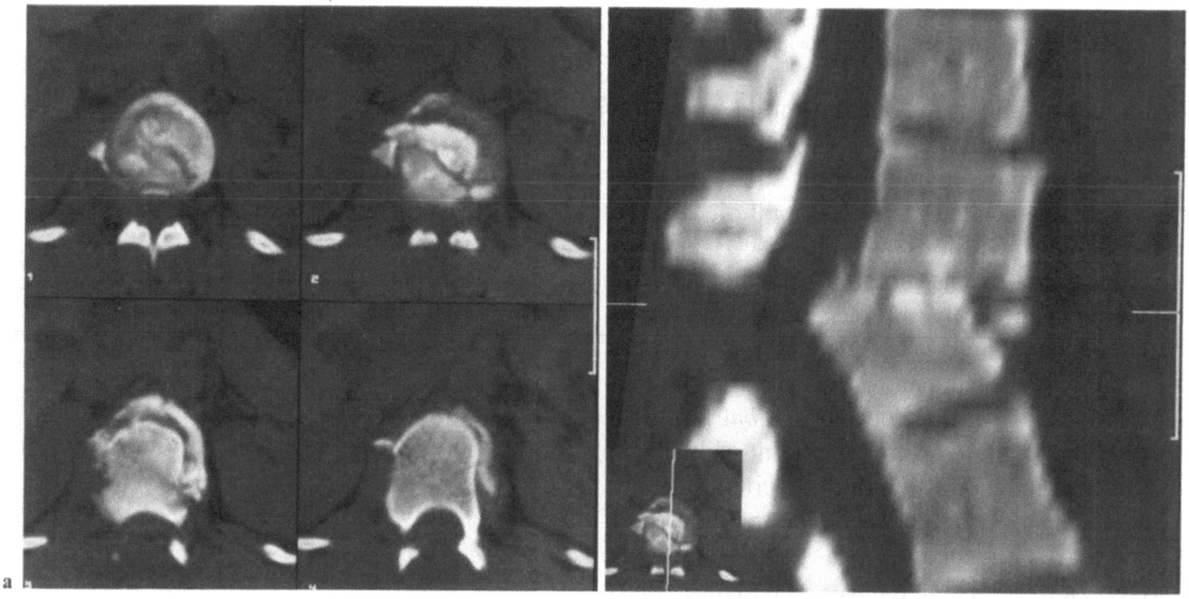

Fig. 48a, b. Flexion-distraction injury. a Contiguous slices of upper part of L1 *(from upper left to lower right)*. Anterior and lateral wedging of upper end-plate. The oblique fracture of the vertebral body does not extend to the base. The naked facets suggest joint disruption. b Mid-sagittal reconstruction shows marked kyphosis, triangular fragment of posterior wall of vertebral body and a smaller fragment of anterior wall. T12 is intact. Gross widening of the interspinous space indicates rupture of supra- and interspinous ligaments

of the spinous processes. The posterior border of the vertebral body is usually longer than the anterior border, producing a wedge shape. The intervertebral space is narrowed. Whereas one of the adjacent vertebral bodies is intact, there is a comminuted fracture of the end-plate of the other.

If the fracture also traverses the posterior border, the spinal canal is narrowed by broken-off fragments. The smaller structures are involved either by dislocation of the articulations or as fractures through the pedicles, pars interarticularis and articular processes.

The AP view is not very characteristic. There is a widening of the interspinous distance. It may be impossible to distinguish between a flexion-distraction fracture and an impression wedge fracture. In the lateral view kyphosis is usually more marked than in wedge or burst fractures.

CT Scan. In contrast to the distraction fracture, the transverse slices show a comminuted fracture of the end-plate of one vertebral body while the adjacent body is intact. The demonstration of a fragment in the spinal canal confirms the involvement of the posterior border and is an important feature. The fracture-line in the pars interarticularis of the arch may be difficult to detect if it runs in the same plane as the CT section. On the other hand, fractures of the articular processes are clearly visible.

Dislocation of small joints produces the sign of the "naked facets".

Sagittal computer reconstructions clarify the comminuted fracture of the end-plate and the intactness of the adjacent vertebra, the angular kyphosis and the splaying of the spinous processes. They are very useful in classifying the fracture (Fig. 48).

VI. Fracture - Dislocation

This designates that group of fractures which exhibit the greatest degree of instability: they are usually unstable in all directions of movement. A common feature is a step-shaped displacement of the spinal canal. McAfee [68] and Magerl [71] call this a "translational injury". But though translation is the commonest mechanism, it is not the only one that may give rise to this injury.

Therefore we prefer with DENIS [19] the term "fracture-dislocation".

The instability is the outcome of destruction of all three columns by very considerable exertion of force, as may be indicated by such frequently observed associated injuries as multiple rib fractures, serial avulsions of transverse or spinous processes or extensive soft tissue damage. The latter may affect the muscles, bowel and parenchymatous organs.

The disko-ligamentous or osteo-disko-ligamentous injury usually develops at *one* level. The direction of the fracture in the individual case depends on the direction of the exerted force and the degree of flexion or torsion at the moment of injury. A severe neurologic lesion is almost the rule. TRAFTON [113] reports 10 patients, all of whom had neurologic deficits, 7 of types A or B in Frankel's classification.

The pattern of injury is not uniform, so that an exact classification may be difficult. Two groups may be distinguished according to the mechanism of injury: a predominantly translational movement with a shear effect and a predominantly rotational movement around the longitudinal axis of the spine.

1. Dislocation

Plain Film. Pure dislocation without bony involvement is very rare. Both anterior and lateral dislocation postulate a rupture of the very tight joint capsules of the facet joints. The lateral view, best as a tomogram, shows the displacement of the upper vertebra over the lower. The dislocated vertebra is tilted slightly caudally, with a corresponding increase in the space between the spinous processes. If the articular processes lie on top of each other, this is a "dislocation on the top" and the intervertebral foramen is widened.

If the articular processes are hooked into each other, this is a "dislocation over the top" and the inferior processes of the dislocated vertebra are projected into the intervertebral foramen.

In the AP view a step in the lateral borders of the vertebral bodies should be looked for. The interpeduncular distance is normal. Frequently, minor decentering of the spinous process indicates an additional rotation.

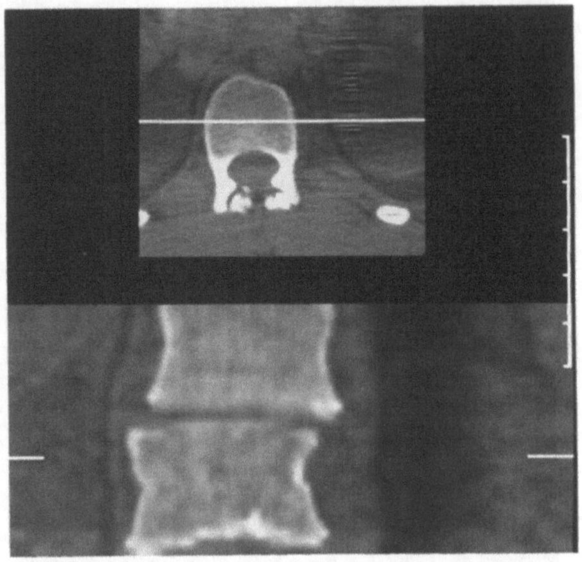

Fig. 49. Translational injury at L1-2. A series of transverse scans showed no fracture of the vertebral bodies, pedicles or laminae. Coronal reconstruction shows shift of the upper vertebra to the left and paravertebral hematoma

CT Scan. CT is particularly indicated if a neurologic deficit cannot be accounted for by the plain films. This occurs most commonly at the cervico-thoracic junction. The transverse slices show the vertebral bodies to be intact. A sudden alteration in position between the dislocated and undislocated vertebrae may be noted in the image, a sign which is quite discrete in a subluxation but very evident in dislocation (Fig. 49).

Without sagittal reconstructions it may be difficult when assessing the articular processes to detect a dislocation on the top. It is possible that the examiner, expecting to find a fracture, may overlook the sign of the naked facet.

In "over the top" dislocation the corresponding joint surfaces seem to be at the normal level, but the half-moon-shaped portions are not turned towards each other but have their convex aspects back to back. The sagittal reconstruction readily clarifies the situation.

2. Fracture-Dislocation

Here we are concerned with a fracture involving the articulations. The effective force is exerted from the dorsal aspect, less often from ventrally. The mechanism is one of shearing. The result is a

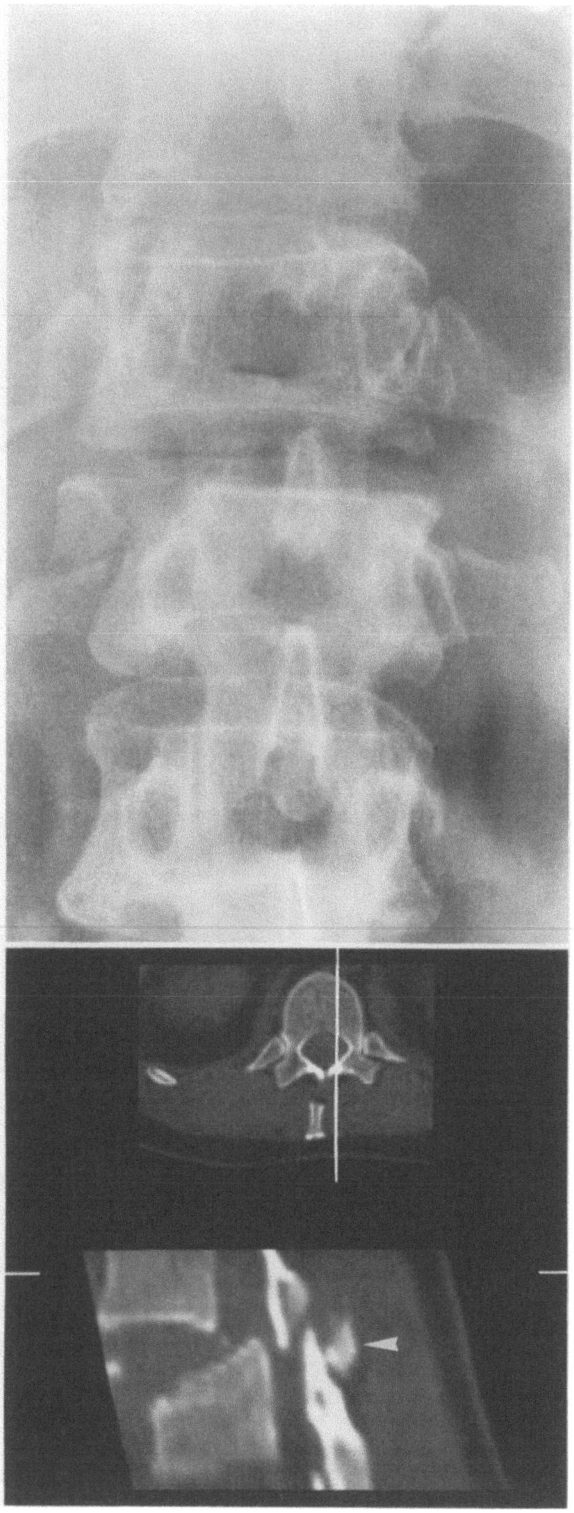

horizontal transection of all three columns with a shift of the upper fragments in the line of force. There are all combinations of bony and disko-ligamentous lesions.

Dorsally, there is either a fracture running through the articular processes or an avulsion fracture of the spinous process or the entire arch at one or two segments. However, in a dorsal dislocation there is no arch fracture.

Plain Film. There is a striking anterior or posterior displacement of one vertebra on the next, with one vertebral body remaining intact. In a dislocation with a kyphotic position a small fragment may sometimes be avulsed from the upper anterior margin of the lower vertebra.

CT Scan. In the discal type, the transverse slices show an intact vertebral body or a small fragment at the anterior border. At the level of dislocation in a postero-anterior type the image of a spondylolisthesis may be obtained; the disk overlaps the posterior margin of the dislocated vertebra posteriorly. If a thick slice has been chosen, a double-lumen sign may also be present. The interruption of the spinal canal is obvious.

It is a simple matter to diagnose an avulsion of the laminae or the spinous process as an obvious cleft can be seen.

The most impressive images are provided by sagittal reconstructions, which best show the dislocated position of the vertebral bodies or fragments and the obstruction of the spinal canal (Figs. 50–52).

Fig. 50 a, b. Postero-anterior type of fracture-dislocation of L1. **a** Antero-posterior view shows double silhouette of upper end-plate, right lateral wedge fracture and bilateral transverse process fractures. **b** Paramedian sagittal reconstruction with reference scan *(upper part)* through T12. No fracture of T12 body or pedicles. Reconstruction shows antelisthesis of T12 on L1, marked narrowing of spinal canal, complete dislocation of articular processes and fracture of "left behind" tip of lower articular process of T12 *(arrowhead)*

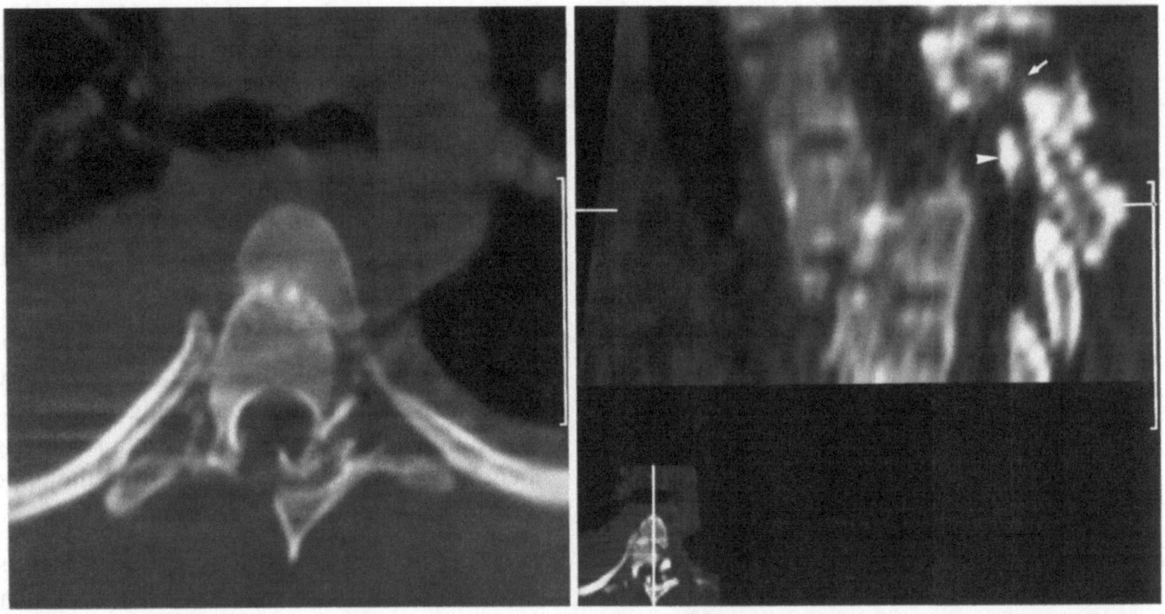

a b

Fig. 51 a, b. Postero-anterior fracture-dislocation at T9–10. **a** Transverse scan shows anterior displacement of vertebral body of T9 on T10. The vertebral arch is torn off and "left behind". Pedicular fractures of T10. Large pleural hematoma. **b** Mid-sagittal reconstruction shows Z-shaped deformation of spinal canal with an indwelling fragment of the posterior arch of T9 *(arrowhead)*. Fracture of articular process *(arrow)*

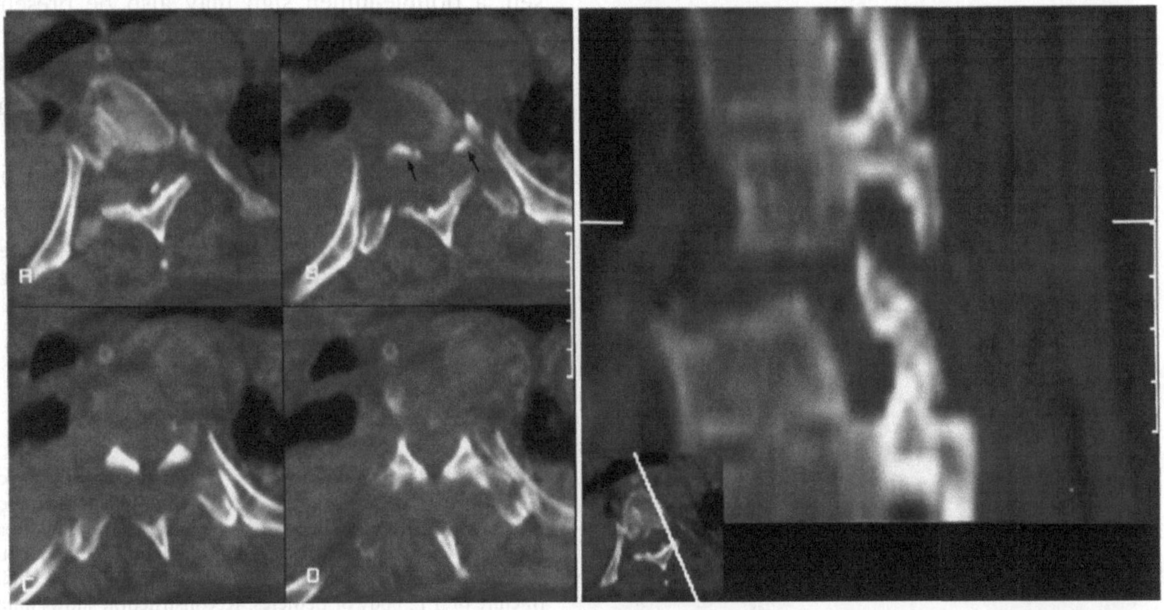

a b

Fig. 52 a, b. Antero-posterior type of fracture-dislocation at T8–9. **a** Four contiguous slices *(upper left to lower right)* beginning at the base of T8 seem to show a widened spinal canal, but note the position of the tips of the articular processes immediately behind the posterior aspect of the vertebral body *(arrows)*. No laminar fracture. **b** Reconstructed oblique images provide better information. Intact articular processes with widened interspinous gap. Retrolisthesis of T8 on T9 obliterates the spinal canal. Widening of the disk space is evidence of rupture

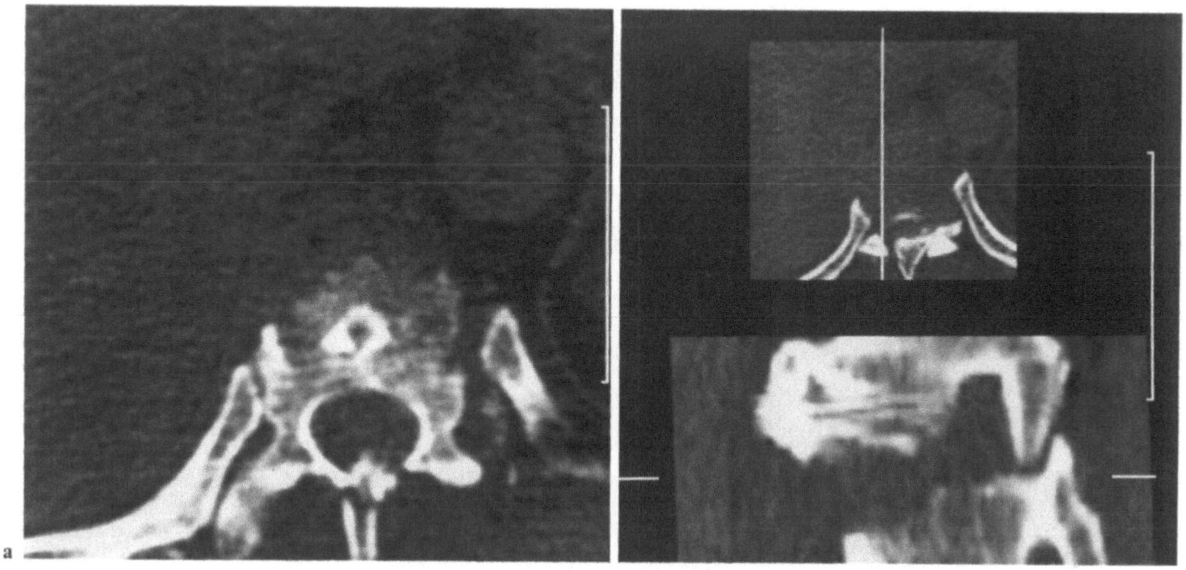

Fig. 53a, b. Slice fracture of T11 in a young man hit in the back by a tree. **a** Transverse scan shows defect of anterior part of vertebral body, fracture of the spinous process and intact pedicles. **b** Parasagittal reconstruction. The reference image *(upper part)* shows absence of the vertebral body, as did some subsequent slices. Reconstructed image *(lower part)* provides clarification: horizontal fracture of vertebral body and part of disk, anterior displacement of T10 and narrowing of spinal canal. Complete dislocation of articular processes without fracture

3. Slice Fracture

This injury is the outcome of a translation associated with rotation; no flexion or axial compression is involved. The fracture-line is altogether horizontal. This is a typical fracture of the thoracolumbar junction. Depending on the degree of shift of the fragment, the fracture may be stable to axial loading but it is unstable to all other forces.

Plain Film. The first feature is the striking horizontal course of the fracture through the vertebral body, with a resulting step-formation in all projections. There is no reduction in vertebral height. Unlike the Chance fracture, there is a step at the anterior and posterior margins as well as a possible rotation between the upper and lower vertebral fragment.

CT Scan. In reviewing the transverse slices from cranially to caudally there is an apparently abrupt discontinuity in the portrayal of the vertebral cuts. This affects both the site of the sagittal and transverse axes.

As the fracture runs horizontally, the fracture gap lies in an unfavorable plane for CT, but the interruption of the spinal canal cannot be missed. A fragment of the articular process can usually be found within the canal.

Computer reconstructions clearly demonstrate the bayonet-type of displacement of the fragments with the resulting steps at the anterior and posterior borders (Fig. 53).

4. Rotational Fracture-Dislocation

In this lesion it is assumed that the shearing force has a strong rotational component, so that the main fracture takes a spiral course. In the individual case this is modified by other factors. Marked flexion (sagittal or lateral) results in a flexion-rotation fracture-dislocation. If there is strong axial compression a rotational burst fracture-dislocation develops.

Plain Film. In the flexion-rotation fracture-dislocation, serial fractures of the ribs or transverse processes can normally be seen in the AP view. The rotation is often also evident. The lateral film likewise shows step formation, which clearly distinguishes this fracture from a Chance fracture.

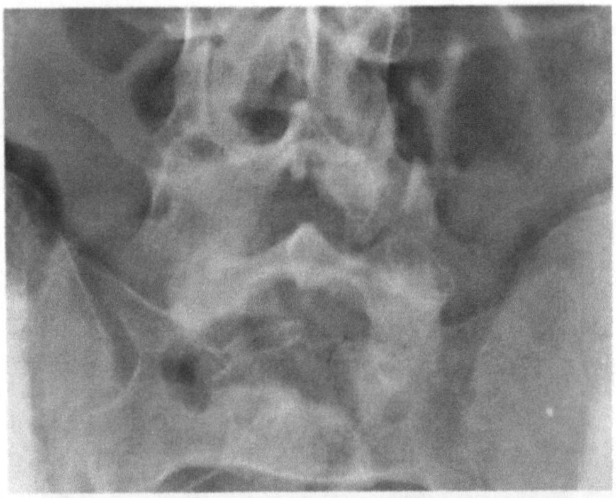
a

Fig. 54 a–c. Flexion-rotation fracture-dislocation at L4–5. **a** AP view shows fracture of left articular pillar of L4 and rotation of L5 to right. **b** Transverse CT cut of L4 shows fracture of left articular pillar, rotation of vertebral body to right side, widening of spinal canal and subluxation of facet joint on right. **c** Transverse cut at L4–5. Part of lower end-plate of L4 on anterior aspect rotated to right. Comminuted fracture of the body of L5 rotated to left. Oblique direction of main fracture line

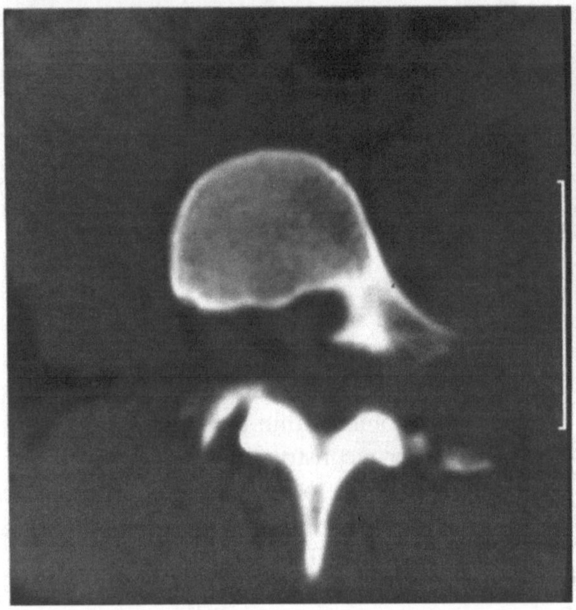
b

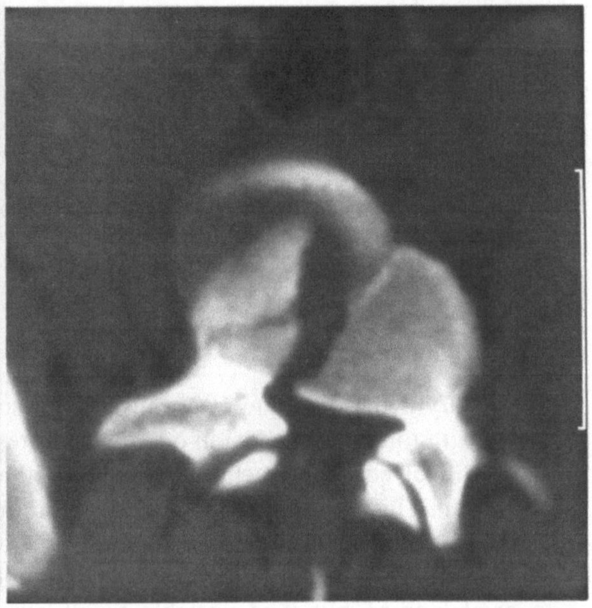
c

The fracture runs diagonally through one or two segments and involves various vertebral components.

In the rotational burst fracture-dislocation the lateral view may resemble a simple burst fracture because the rotation is unrecognized. On the other hand, the step formation in the frontal plane is immediately spotted in the AP view and the main fracture-line runs towards the long axis somewhat diagonally. The damaged vertebra is reduced in height to a varying extent. The upper segments can be seen to be rotated in relation to the lower, which further contributes to the lateral step formation.

The fractures of the transverse processes are very characteristic. In the classic case they are situated together with the fracture-line of the vertebral body on a spiral curve. Cranial to the fractured vertebra, they are found on the side to which the vertebral fracture extends cranially; below, they lie on the opposite side.

The injuries to the joints also correspond to the oblique course of the fracture. On the side where the force is applied (i.e. where the vertebral body fracture begins cranially) there is a dislocation, whereas on the opposite side there is a fracture of the isthmus or the articular processes.

CT Scan. The major injuries require the display of at least two segments; the minor ones are sometimes evident in 5 or more segments. It is also advantageous in these complicated fractures

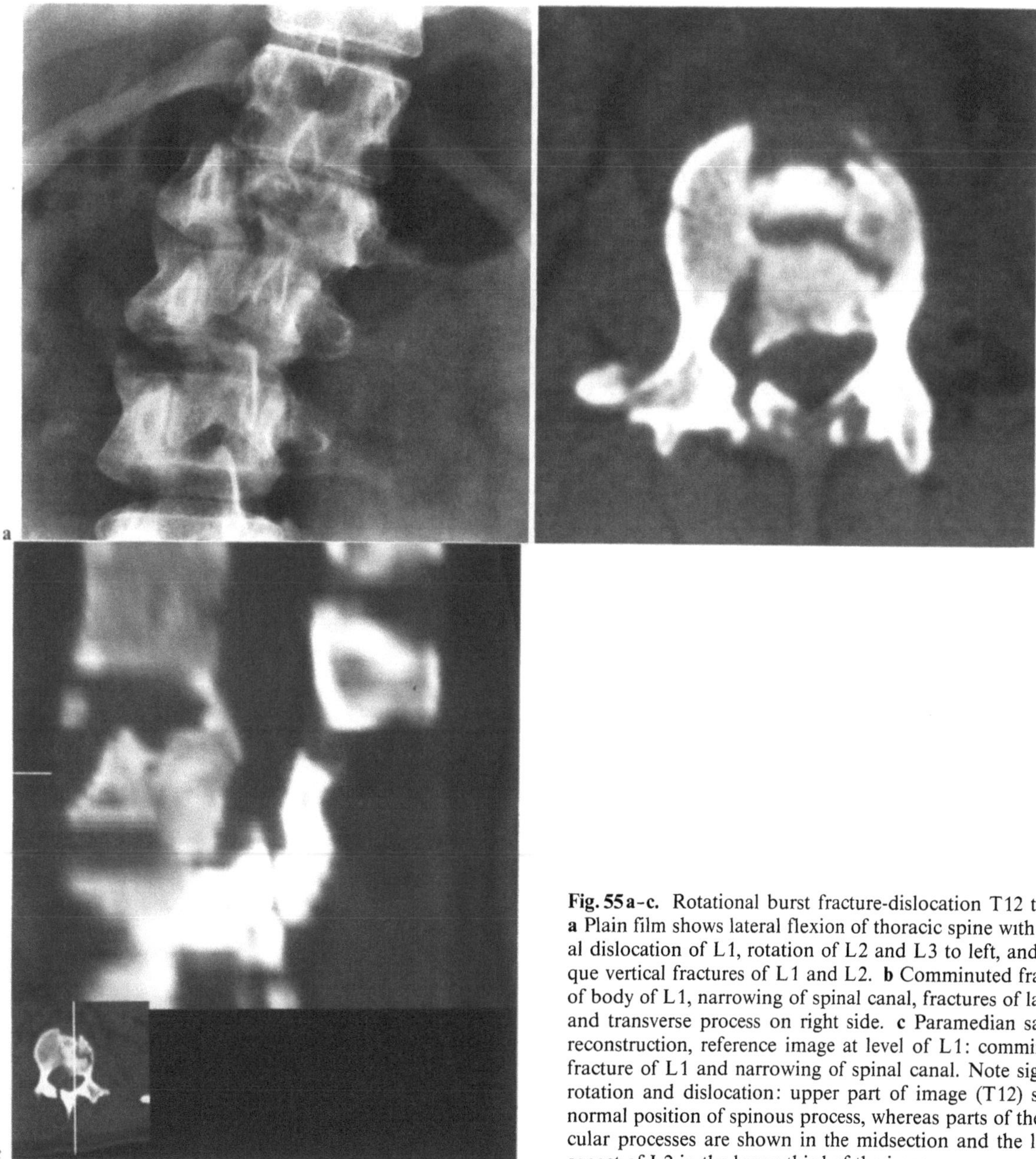

Fig. 55 a–c. Rotational burst fracture-dislocation T12 to L2. **a** Plain film shows lateral flexion of thoracic spine with lateral dislocation of L1, rotation of L2 and L3 to left, and oblique vertical fractures of L1 and L2. **b** Comminuted fracture of body of L1, narrowing of spinal canal, fractures of lamina and transverse process on right side. **c** Paramedian sagittal reconstruction, reference image at level of L1: comminuted fracture of L1 and narrowing of spinal canal. Note signs of rotation and dislocation: upper part of image (T12) shows normal position of spinous process, whereas parts of the articular processes are shown in the midsection and the lateral aspect of L2 in the lower third of the image

to make continuous sections and first consider them in sequence. This is the quickest way to note the step formation and faulty rotation of the vertebra, the break in the spinal canal as well as the fractured ribs and transverse processes. In addition, posterior wall fragments may also present though this is not an essential feature.

Denis [20] points out that the distinguishing feature of the burst fracture is that the posterior longitudinal ligament remains intact, whereas it is torn in the flexion-rotation fracture-dislocation.

There is no difficulty in recognizing the instability of the fracture. Further evidence of the destruction of the posterior column is the unilateral joint dislocation and the contralateral joint fracture.

As the fracture runs obliquely through the vertebral body, the fracture gap "wanders" from image to image. Depending on the degree of bayonet-type step formation, laterally from the still intact upper vertebra fragments of the lower vertebra can be distinguished. If the position of the spinous processes is compared it is simple to note the different rotation.

The facet joint is dislocated on the side of the impact. Contralaterally, the fracture usually traverses the inferior articular process of the upper vertebra and the superior process of the lower. Arch fractures likewise tend to be situated on this side.

In the rotational burst fracture the vertebral body is split into several fragments, also involving the posterior margin. This narrows the spinal canal, if it has not been completely interrupted by the dislocation.

As a rule, several computed reconstructions are needed to display the full extent of the situation. Because of the rotation and dislocation, many images will show only part of the spine depending on the site of the reconstructed slice. Sagittal computed reconstructions visualize the malalignment and the kyphosis and confirm the interruption of the spinal canal with the intrusion of bony fragments (Figs. 54, 55).

Chapter 3 Injuries of the Intervertebral Disk and Neural Tissues

A. Injuries of the Intervertebral Disk

Traumatic disk herniations are found in 3% to 30% of spinal injuries [47, 53, 75, 111]. They may be seen in association with fractures, dislocations, gunshot wounds or without any associated injury ("isolated traumatic disk herniation") and may be the source of neurologic deficits [93].

The intervertebral disks are rarely affected by a direct penetrating injury. Injuries of the disks are rather caused by indirect trauma.

Rupture of the disk can be evoked by two different mechanisms: flexion and extension, both combined with a rotational component.

The intervertebral disk is quite resistant to excessive pressure forces [85, 106]. In compression injuries, a fracture of the vertebra usually occurs before a nondegenerated disk is crushed. This explains why compression fractures of the vertebrae are most frequently encountered in regions with a heavy axial load, whereas compressive intervertebral disk injuries occur mainly at levels with a high prevalence of degenerative changes, that is to say in the lower cervical and lower lumbar regions. A fragment of the nucleus can be extruded by axial compression and can penetrate through tears and disintegrated parts of the anulus fibrosus. Trauma in these cases is rather the occasion than the causative factor of a disk herniation that would have happened anyway [58].

Traction experiments have demonstrated a relatively high degree of vulnerability of the disk. In traction strains the intervertebral disk is damaged before the adjacent vertebra suffers any injury. Isolated traumatic disk herniation may occur following distraction. Traction forces are typical in hyperextension and hyperflexion injuries and in lateral inclination of the spine. Under traction forces, the disk ruptures near the cartilaginous end-plate. Disk fragments can be extruded from the intervertebral space.

Ruptures of the intervertebral disks are a common finding in fractures of the spine. Especially, severe dislocations of the vertebrae are possible only in association with a severe injury of the involved disk [106]. Fractures of the vertebral end-plates are often associated with tears of the fibrocartilaginous anulus fibrosus. In vertebral fractures, the gelatinous material of the nucleus pulposus or even part of the anulus fibrosus can thus penetrate between the fragments of the vertebral body. Most herniated disks caused by cervical trauma remain anterior to the posterior longitudinal ligament and can thus be excised through an anterior operative approach [5].

Traumatic disk herniation can be diagnosed by CT. The CT appearance of isolated traumatic disk herniation is the same as that of herniation unrelated to trauma [79]. This includes soft tissue densities abutting the ventral or lateral portion of the spinal canal or intervertebral foramen, sometimes associated with gas or calcifications (Figs. 56, 58).

The need to use an intrathecal contrast medium in traumatic disk herniation is being obviated by MRI. The advantage of MRI is better tissue contrast that allows for assessment of ligamentous structures, especially the anterior and posterior longitudinal ligaments (Figs. 57, 58).

One further benefit of MRI is its lack of artifacts in the cervicothoracic region and the demonstration of concomitant spinal cord compression, epidural and subligamentous hematoma [51, 53, 111]. MRI is ideal for evaluating trauma to the disk and adjacent structures. Disk pathology and herniation into the spinal canal associated with ligamentous rupture are clearly seen [70]. MRI can even distinguish disk hemorrhage from disk degeneration [75].

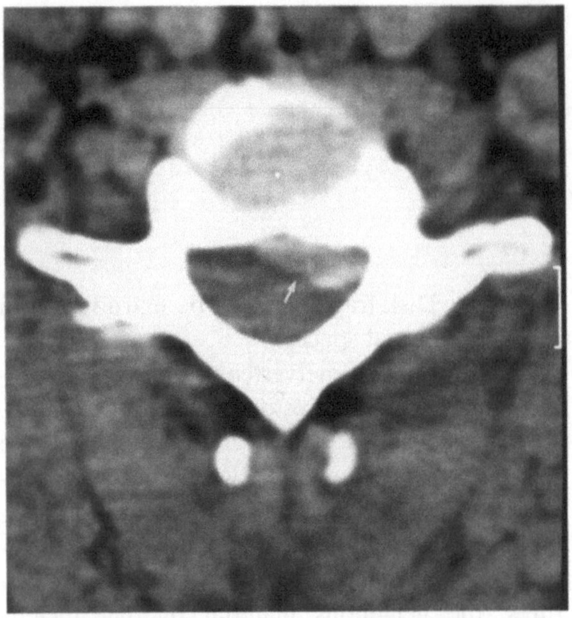

Fig. 56. CT scan of a traumatic medio-lateral disk herniation at C5/C6 *(arrow)*. Attenuation value of the disk *(white point)* 93 HU; very similar values were measured in the herniated part

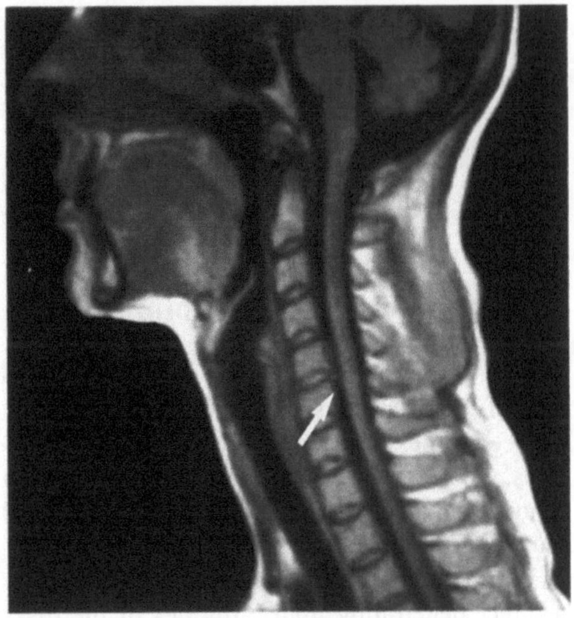

Fig. 57. T1-weighted sagittal MRI scan of a traumatic disk herniation *(arrow)* at C5/C6. Note the absence of disk degeneration and of vertebral fracture

a
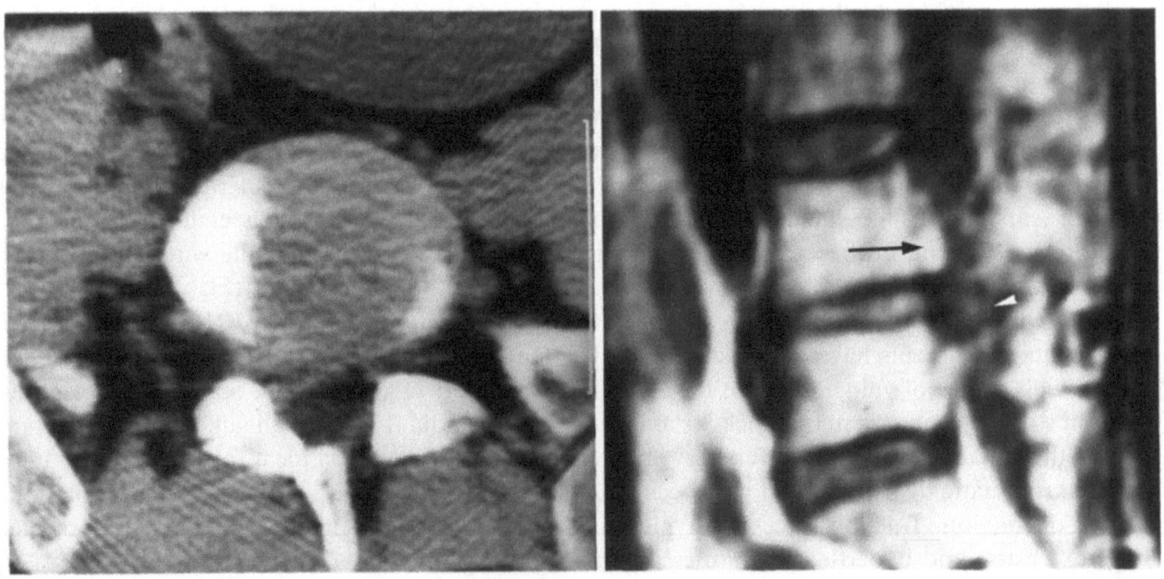
b

Fig. 58 a, b. Traumatic disk herniation at L4/L5. **a** Axial CT shows medio-lateral herniation indistinguishable from disk degeneration. **b** Sagittal T1-weighted MRI demonstrates diminished height of the disk, a small amount of the herniated material (most of it was lateral) in the spinal canal *(arrowhead)* and a concomitant retrovertebral hematoma *(arrow)* as a high intensity structure

B. Accompanying Injuries of the Neural Tissues and Their Coverings

I. Dura Mater

In traumatic leaks through the dura mater, CT after intrathecal injection of contrast medium is the method of choice [77]. Dural tears can be demonstrated by conventional myelography. However, myelography may be undesirable because the necessary patient manipulations can aggravate or produce neurologic deficits. Moreover, myelography alone may fail to show minor extravasations of cerebrospinal fluid (CSF) and contrast medium. A noncontrast CT scan can also demonstrate only relatively large CSF collections as lesions isodense to water. CT-myelography, on the other hand, is able to show even small amounts of CSF extravasation beyond the normal confines of the thecal sac, the site of the dural tear, herniation of nerve-roots through the defect and a possible nerve-root or cauda equina entrapment in the tear or in bony fragments [93].

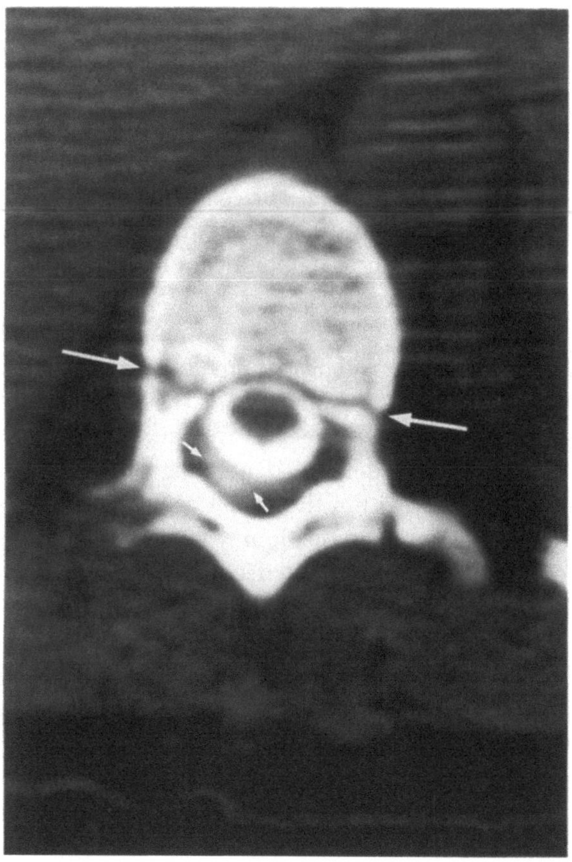

Fig. 59. Dural laceration with formation of a pseudomeningocele *(small arrows)* following bilateral fracture *(large arrows)* of the pedicles of T12. Myelo-CT

If the torn dura heals, there may result pouches of CSF beyond the confines of the thecal sac, so-called pseudomeningoceles. The nerve-roots may become entrapped in these cavities [77] (Fig. 59).

II. Nerve-root Avulsion

Avulsion of a nerve or nerve-root sleeve is usually accompanied by a dural laceration following a stretching injury to an extremity [93]. Most often it follows an injury of the shoulder. The intraspinal nerve-root is separated from the spinal cord and a cuff of dura-arachnoid is usually avulsed from the thecal sac as well. Retraction of the nerve stump creates a cavity that is later filled with CSF. This pseudomeningocele can be demonstrated radiographically [48, 93].

Nerve-root avulsion in the cervical spine commonly occurs in the lower cervical and first thoracic segments. CT-myelography demonstrates pseudomeningoceles with extension of the expanded nerve-root sleeves through the neural foramina. The contrast medium extravasates into fascial planes between the anterior and middle scalenus muscles towards the brachial plexus region. CT, because of its superior spatial resolution, is so far unsurpassed in assessing even minute changes such as deficiency of the anterior or posterior root within the subarachnoid space. This may be the case even without pseudomeningocele formation.

If fibrosis, scarring and arachnoidal adhesions are associated with an avulsion, then the contrast-enhanced CT scan may fail to show a contrast-filled pseudomeningocele but an extradural defect is seen instead [93]. Congenital elongation of cervical root pouches and lateral meningoceles associated with spinal neurofibromatosis can be differential diagnoses in nerve-root avulsion.

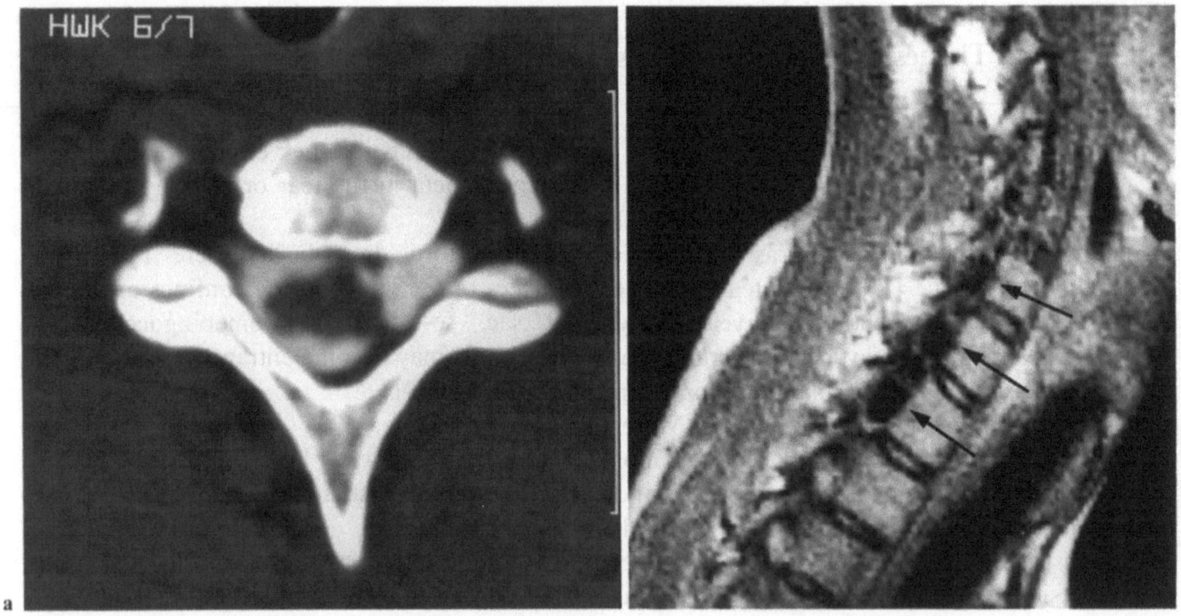

Fig. 60 a, b. Avulsion of left brachial plexus. **a** CT-myelography at C6/C7 demonstrates pseudomeningocele formation and absence of the ventral and dorsal roots. **b** Sagittal T1-weighted MRI shows lack of epidural fat and neural structures in the intervertebral foramina involved *(arrows)*. CSF-equivalent low signal intensity is seen instead ("empty foramen sign")

Myelography may fail to show the avulsion within the first weeks following trauma [64]. CT in the acute stage demonstrates obliteration by hemorrhage of the soft tissue structures in the intervertebral foramen (spinal nerve and ganglion, fat). As the spinal nerves are invested with epidural venous plexuses, nerve-root avulsion can produce an epidural hematoma [93]. Avulsion of the nerve-roots from the spinal cord in one of our cases led to spinal subarachnoid hemorrhage.

Pseudomeningoceles of the cervical dura are readily visualized by MRI. In the T1-weighted image, they appear as hypointense fluid collections in the region of the intervertebral foramen. On the T2-weighted scan the signal intensity is high accordingly. In pseudomeningoceles, the content of the intervertebral foramina is abnormal: adipose tissue and neural structures are replaced by CSF-isointense material. This "empty foramen sign" should be remembered especially in assessing sagittal scans (Fig. 60).

Due to its reduced spatial resolution, MRI in our experience is as yet unable to completely substitute CT-myelography. Obscure nerve-root pathology is prone to be overlooked on MRI alone.

III. Epidural Hematoma

Spinal epidural hematomas due to trauma are relatively uncommon. They can result from severe or minimal trauma. They may even develop spontaneously or as a complication of anticoagulant therapy. As the epidural space in the spine contains mainly veins, these epidural hematomas seldom present such a dramatic clinical picture as their cranial counterparts. Neurologically, these lesions may cause severe pain and increasing neurologic deficits, depending on their level and location within the spinal canal. Paraplegia, tetraplegia or even death may occur in rare cases unless rapid surgical decompression is performed in these cases.

The most common area involved is the thoracic spine with its prominent epidural space [83]. Epidural hematomas of the cervical spine have mainly been described as acute lesions, as opposed to those in the lumbar spine which may be chronic [63, 118]. Most spinal epidural hematomas, if not operated upon, will resolve spontaneously over a period of time.

On the axial CT scan, the clotted blood of an epidural spinal hematoma usually appears as a

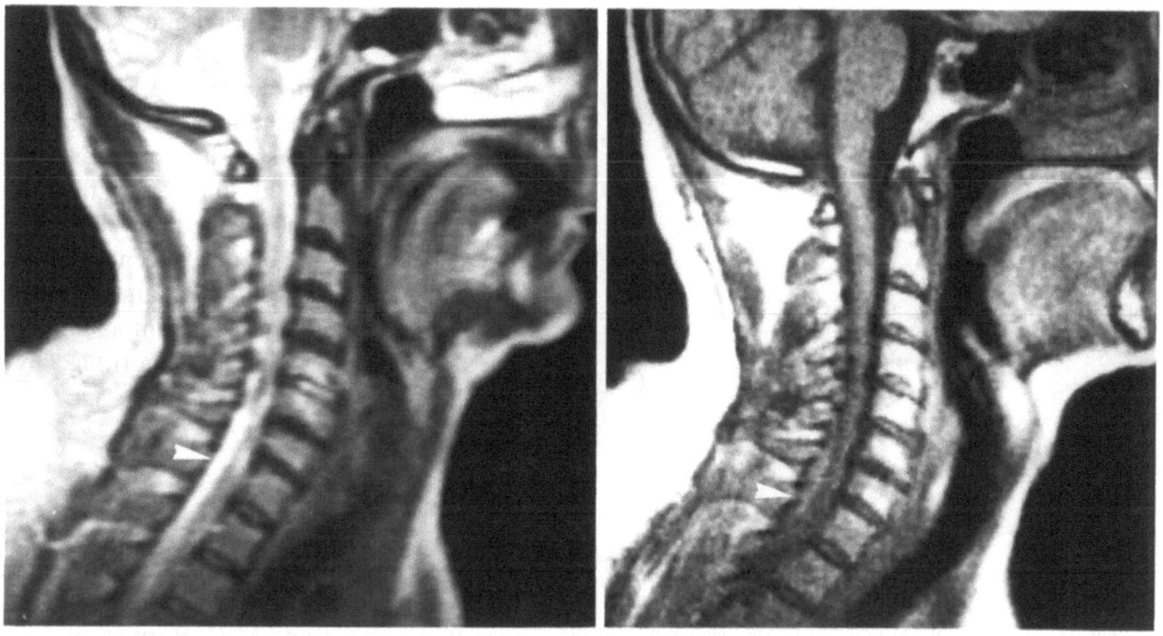

Fig. 61 a, b. Epidural hematoma. a T2-weighted MRI. b T1-weighted image. Both show increased density in the dorsal epidural space at the cervico-thoracic junction *(arrowheads)*

hyperdense mass outlining the bony spinal canal and replacing the epidural adipose tissue. The shape is typically biconvex to circumferential and sharply demarcated [92].

In critical areas (cervicothoracic region) an epidural hematoma and spinal cord compression may be impossible to discern without intrathecal contrast. Intrathecal contrast medium may also be necessary in patients with a discrepancy between the clinical and CT or radiographic findings.

Traumatic or spontaneous disk herniation may be a differential diagnosis. However, unlike herniations, epidural hematomas are not confined to the level of the disk space but rather extend over a considerable distance [92].

On MRI, the appearance of epidural hematomas depends on their age. They should be most obvious within the first week, when their lack of intensity contrasts more with the bright epidural fat. As the hematoma ages, the hemorrhage signal intensity increases due to methemoglobin production and the increased signal may be masked by the fat. The mass effect, however, persists [70].

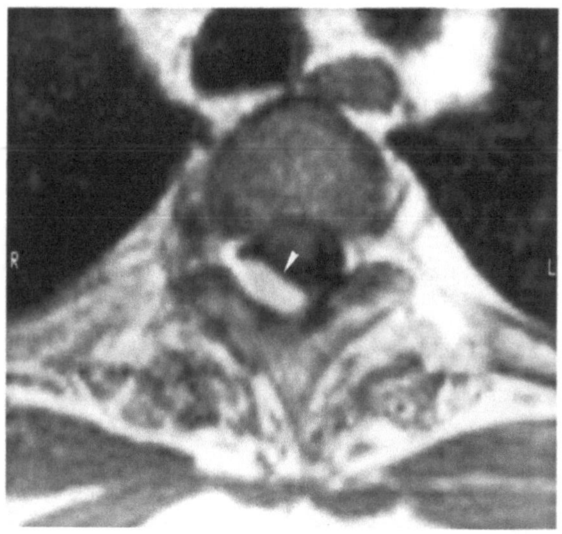

Fig. 62. Subacute thoracic epidural hematoma. Transverse T1-weighted MRI. Hematoma appears as hyperintense space-occupying lesion at the dorsolateral aspect of the spinal canal *(arrowhead)*. Distortion of the spinal cord allows differentiation from normal epidural adipose tissue

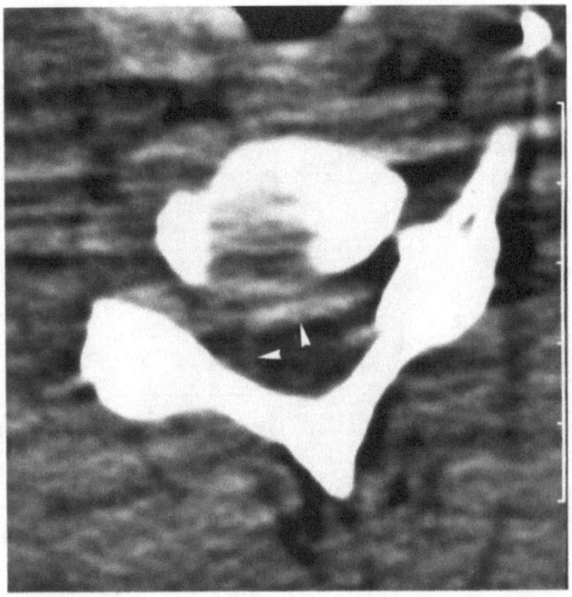

Fig. 63. Avulsion of the brachial plexus. Hematoma in the right intervertebral foramen. Subarachnoid hematoma around the cord mimicks intrathecal contrast medium *(arrowheads)*

IV. Subarachnoid Hemorrhage

Spinal subarachnoid hemorrhage may be associated with other hematomas or nerve-root avulsions. On a plain CT scan it appears as a hyperdense ring encircling the spinal cord, thus resembling intrathecal contrast medium. This appearance depends on the blood concentration in the CSF. Unless there is a sufficient amount of blood in the subarachnoid space, it is impossible to detect a spinal subarachnoid hemorrhage by CT [93].

V. Soft Tissues

Soft tissue hematoma and ligamentous ruptures can be suspected from effacement of soft and adipose tissue on CT and MRI. Rupture of the supportive ligaments is not an uncommon finding on MRI [70]. The ruptures of the normally hypointense dark ligaments can already be imaged within the first week following trauma. Sagittal views are best to evaluate ruptures of the longitudinal ligaments, ligamentum flavum, and inter- and supraspinous ligaments (Figs. 64, 68, and 69).

a

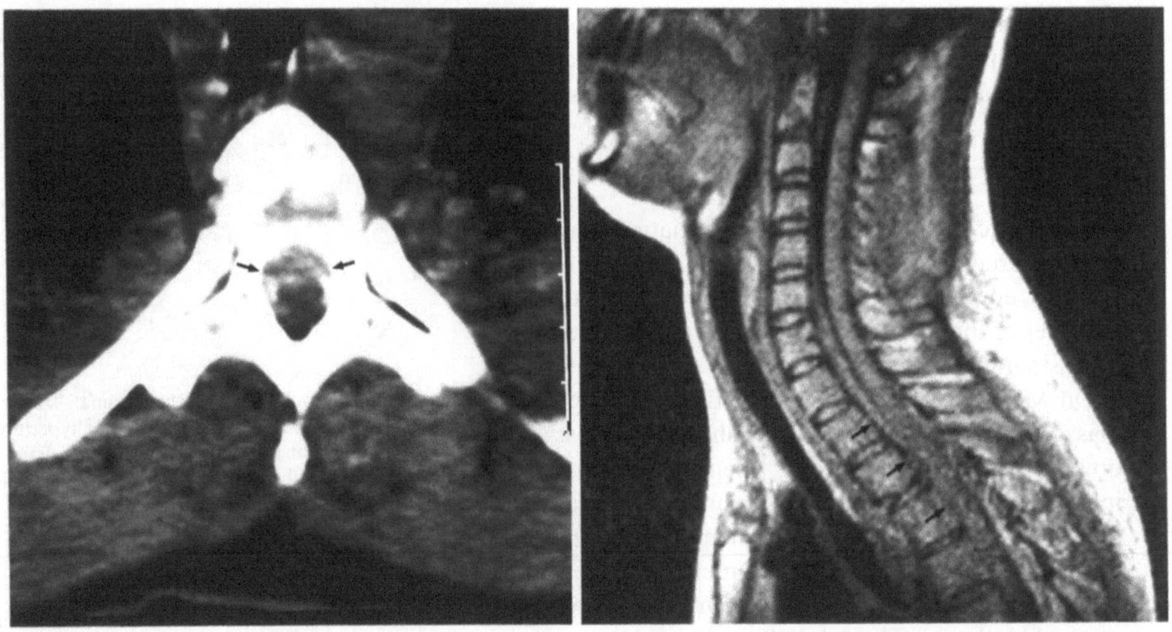

b

Fig. 64 a, b. Subligamentous hematoma above a thoracic vertebral fracture (T7, not shown). **a** CT-myelography at the level T4/T5 demonstrates epidural space-occupying lesion *(arrows)*. **b** Sagittal MRI (T1-weighted) shows cranio-caudal extension of the hematoma effacing the epidural space *(arrows)*

Lesions of the ligaments of the cranio-cervical junction play an essential role. The integrity of the transverse atlantal ligament can be assessed even on the basis of conventional lateral radiographs. A distance between the odontoid and the posterior aspect of the anterior atlantal arch greater than 3 mm indicates a lesion of the ligament.

Assessment of the alar ligaments requires special CT examinations. The alar ligaments extend from the dens to the occipital condyles and act so as to restrict lateral head rotation. Their rupture has been shown to be frequent, with an incidence of 30% in autopsy series [103]. Measurement of the segmental rotatory movement by CT can be employed to support diagnosis of occipitoaxial hypermobility and probable rupture of the alar ligaments [25, 26].

VI. Spinal Cord

Lacerations of the cord are rare. They are seen in association with very severe impact in a transverse shearing, flexion-rotation or direct injury. Direct spinal cord trauma with injury of the dura mater (stabbing, gunshot wounds) represents only a minority of cases (Fig. 65).

The vast majority consists of blunt spinal cord injuries. Four stages can be distinguished in the traumatized cord [49].

1. Early stage: hemorrhage and necrosis
2. Intermediate stage: resorption and organization
3. End stage: scarring, secondary tract degeneration
4. Epiphenomena: syrinx formation, microcystic myelomalacia.

Injury to the cord is most commonly located at the lower cervical cord and thoracolumbar region. Concomitant spinal stenosis increases the danger of traumatic spinal cord damage. The greatest transverse extent of pathoanatomic changes is at the epicenter of the traumatic forces. There is, however, a marked tendency to craniocaudal spread of microcirculatory and metabolic damage along the spinal axis with several segments being involved [64]. Hemor-

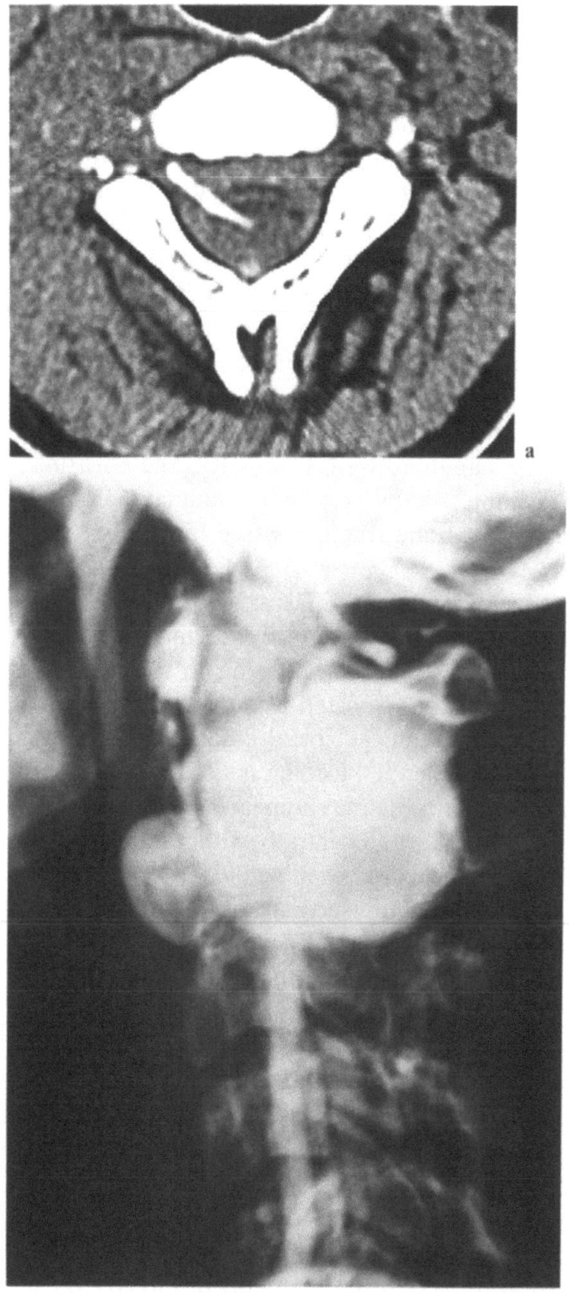

a

b

Fig. 65 a, b. Direct cord injury by a glass splinter at C2/C3 in a young woman who fell backward through a glass door. No severe injury of the skin or soft tissues. Two weeks later she noticed paraesthesia of the 4th and 5th fingers on the right. **a** Transverse high resolution CT scan at the base of C2 shows glass splinter which must have penetrated through the right intervertebral foramen. No immediate surgery because of local skin infection. **b** Angiogram of the right vertebral artery 10 days later, when the patient observered a swelling of the side of the neck. A false aneurysm was resected with protection by balloon occlusion. Uneventful outcome, no neurologic deficit

rhages in the subarachnoid, epidural or subdural spaces are not uncommon, but unlike intracranial lesions they usually have no dramatic space-occupying character.

Crucial pathophysiologic processes after acute spinal cord trauma occur during the first minutes and hours. They generally begin in the central gray matter and proceed with enormous inherent dynamics. At the cord surface, even at the site of traumatic impact, only minor hemorrhages show with a tendency to confluence and spontaneous resolution.

Cord compression and impingement can readily be diagnosed by CT or MRI. The cord may be compressed by hematoma, traumatic disk herniation or bone fragments (see Figs. 56, 58, and 61).

Myelography and CT scanning can be used in the evaluation of spinal cord edema. In patients with edema there is a little or no subarachnoid space anterior or posterior to the cord.

Hematoma in the spinal cord becomes visible on CT only if the bleeding is acute and of sufficient quantity. It may appear as a focal hyperdense area located centrally within the cord with concomitant cord swelling [93]. Cord fissures, laceration and transection are difficult to assess on plain CT.

Large lacerations of the spinal cord may be readily recognized on CT after intrathecal injection of contrast medium. They appear as collections of contrast medium within the cord. In laceration there is rapid passage of contrast medium into the cord. Absence of the cord shadow on plain or contrast CT is seen in cases with severe trauma. These findings probably indicate disruption of the cord anatomy, possibly true cord transection [16, 93]. MRI is capable of directly visualizing cord transection, which may be documented by complete loss of the spinal cord signal [53].

The MRI appearance of other spinal cord trauma is difficult to assess, especially as the aspect of hematomas depends not only on magnetic field strength but also on the age of a hematoma [51].

MRI is rather insensitive in detecting very recent hematomas as relaxation times overlap with gray or white matter. However, it neatly demonstrates focal cord swelling and cord deformity.

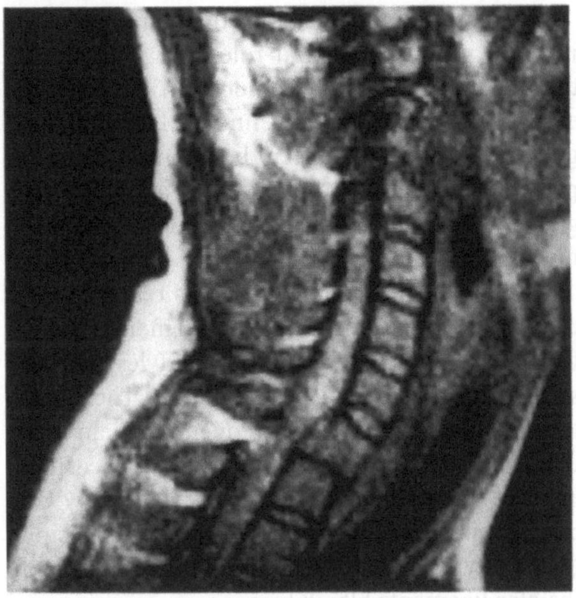

Fig. 66. Paraplegic patient with fracture-dislocation at C7/T1. Sagittal T1-weighted MR image shows increased signal intensity and diffuse swelling of the lower cervical cord. Diagnosis: hemorrhagic cord contusion

Increased signal in a T1-weighted scan is believed to represent methemoglobin formation in a hemorrhagic component [111].

The sensitivity of MRI in detecting cord hematoma increases with time, particularly within the first three days after bleeding has occurred. In the acute phase T1 and T2 are relatively long with a high spin density, and hematoma cannot be differentiated from edema. Shortening of T1 subsequently results within a few days in better contrast between hyperintense hematoma and hypointense edema on T1-weighted images. This change in appearance commences at the periphery of the hematoma and spreads centrally.

In the animal model, high signal intensity on a long spin-echo (SE) sequence was shown to represent edema or necrosis, whereas acute hemorrhage appeared as an area of low intensity in long SE sequences, probably owing to intracellular desoxyhemoglobin [39]. Recent hematoma was about isointense to the cord in short SE sequences. Necrosis and edema could not be distinguished by MRI.

These findings correspond with clinical observations, where subacute spinal hemorrhage was

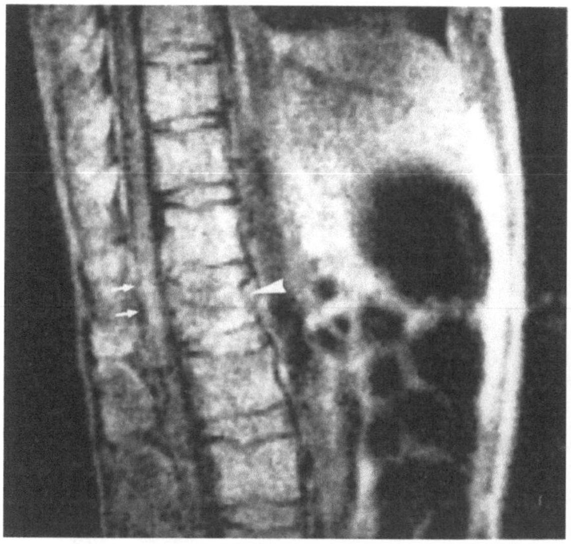

Fig. 67. Sagittal T1-weighted MR image. Patient with burst fracture of T12 *(arrowhead)*. Increased signal intensity in the cord represents hemorrhage *(arrows)*

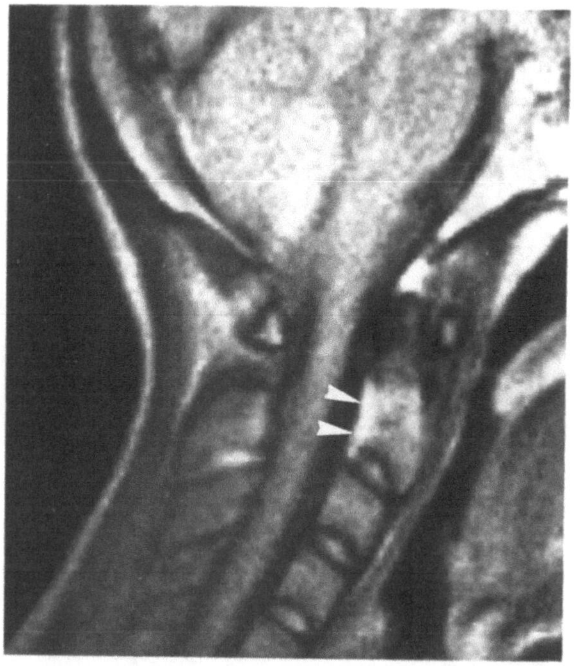

Fig. 68. Fracture of the arch of the axis (same patient as in Figs. 16 and 21). Sagittal T1-weighted MRI. Subacute hemorrhage at the fracture site is indicated by circumscribed hyperintensity *(arrowheads)*. No hemorrhage of the cord

found to present a low signal on T2-weighted images within 3 days after the injury. Cord edema and necrosis on the other hand had a high signal intensity [117].

Kulkarni et al. [59] describe three patterns of spinal cord injury:

1. The most common pattern consists of hyperintensity within the cord on T2-weighted images in the acute phase. The lesions show rapid resolution and the patients experience significant neurologic recovery. The lesions are interpreted as cord edema, possibly associated with petechial hemorrhages.
2. The second pattern involves central hypointensity on T2-weighted images in the subacute stage, evolving into a peripheral rim of hyperintensity with a persistent central area of hypointensity. This pattern is thought to indicate cord hematoma and is associated with the severest neurologic deficits without clinical improvement.
3. The third pattern is a combination of 1) and 2): a central hypointensity on T2-weighted images surrounded by a hyperintense zone. This is believed to represent hemorrhage and surrounding edema.

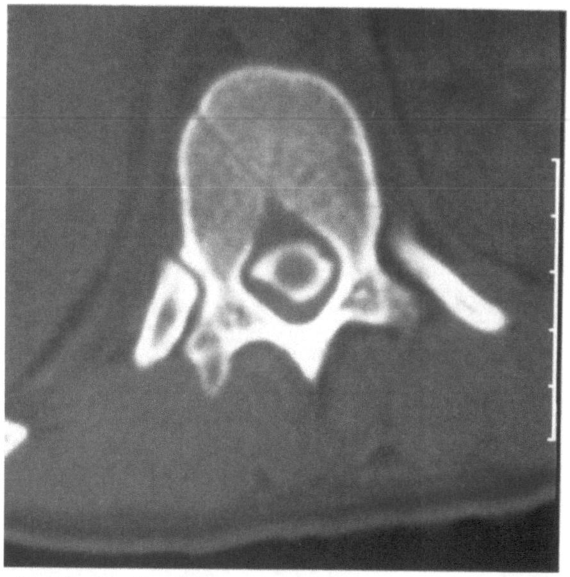

Fig. 69. Small subligamentous hematoma. CT-myelography at the upper upper level of T12 shows circumscribed space-occupying lesion at the dorso-lateral aspect. No fracture

T2-weighted images are useful in the detection not only of spinal cord pathology but also of vertebral body hemorrhage (see Fig. 42) and bleeding along the ligaments that appear as areas of increased signal intensity [60].

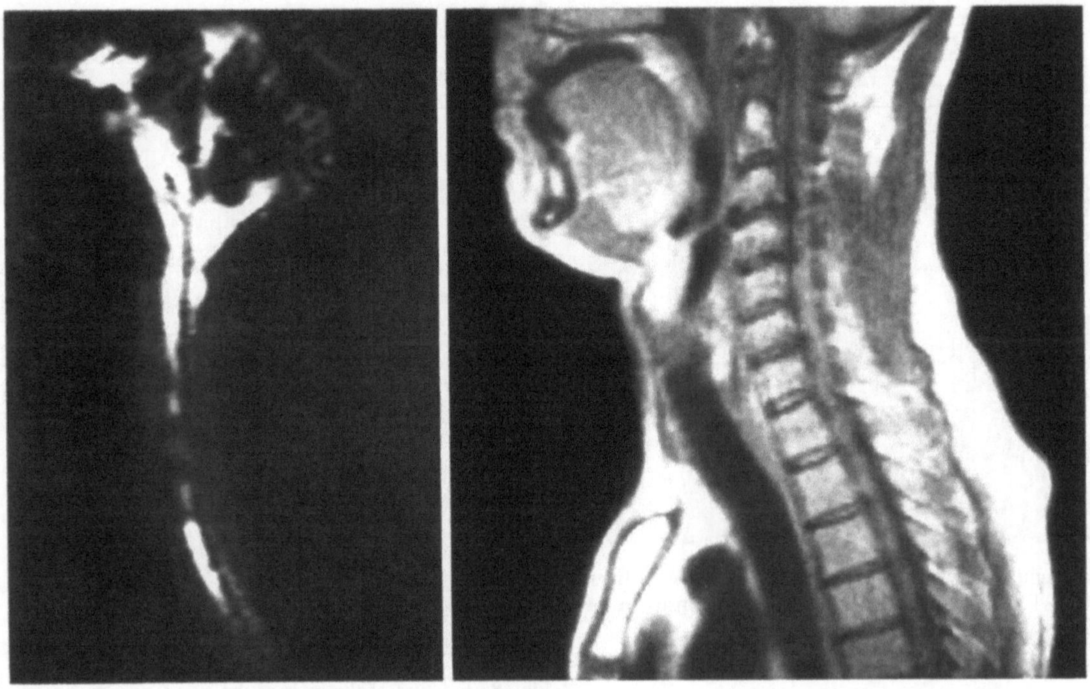

a b

Fig. 70 a, b. Central cord syndrome following a hyperextension injury in a patient with spinal stenosis. **a** Extremely T2-weighted sagittal MRI shows severe narrowing of the subarachnoid space from C3 through C7. **b** T1-weighted image demonstrates increased signal intensity of the cord

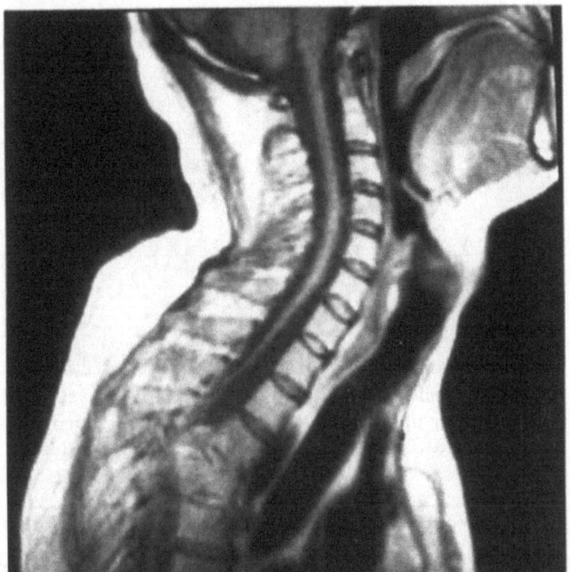

Fig. 71. Severe cord atrophy after flexion-distraction injury at T3/T4. T1-weighted sagittal MRI. Complete spastic paraplegia

Among traumatic cervical spinal cord injuries as a whole there is a subpopulation with little or no radiographic abnormality, except for severe spondylosis or a constitutional spinal stenosis, yet with a profound neurologic deficit [99]. The patients suffer from an acute central cervical cord syndrome. The injuries can be attributed to a narrow spinal canal that makes the cord more susceptible to compression by the ligamenta flava during hyperextension. MRI is the method of choice as it is able to demonstrate noninvasively not only the degree of spinal stenosis but also preexistent chronic damage to the cervical spinal cord.

Posttraumatic atrophy of the spinal cord can be recognized in either MRI or CT by the reduced size of the cord. Atrophy may be focal or, more frequently, a more or less uniformly small spinal cord extends over several segments [79]. It may be associated with a syrinx.

Of the late posttraumatic changes, those deserve special interest that are responsible for what is called "progressive posttraumatic myelopathy". This well-recognized clinical entity has a prevalence of 3% among spinal cord-injured patients. It presents clinically as delayed neurologic deterioration [67].

a) The most common cause of progressive posttraumatic myelopathy is posttraumatic syringomyelia with cyst formation. Posttraumatic spinal cord cysts may be multiple. They are most frequently found in the dorsal portion of the cord and may vary along their length in width and position within the cord [96]. MRI is the method of choice in evaluating the formation of a cyst or syrinx and obviates the need for intrathecal contrast medium and delayed CT scanning, which has a sensitivity of little more than 50% [33, 76, 108]. On MRI the cysts have a signal intensity characteristic of cerebrospinal fluid. They are best demonstrated on a sagittal scanning plane, although small eccentric cavities may be obscured by partial volume averaging [90].

Unlike hydromyelia, which by definition is a dilatation of the central canal, syringomyelia develops eccentric to the canal although it often communicates with it. Usually the cavities are not lined by ependyma. Posttraumatic syringomyelia manifests as cord dilatation above the site of compression [80].

Atypical syringomyelia exists, with cysts containing a viscous fluid that has relaxation times similar to the surrounding neural tissue. Cystic tumor may be a differential diagnosis [90].

b) Posttraumatic arachnoiditis is believed to play a role in posttraumatic progressive myelopathy, inasmuch as there seems to be some influence on microcystic cord degeneration. Arachnoidal adhesions may envelop the spinal cord and lead to severe tethering. Releasing these adhesions may be followed by clinical improvement [67].

Myelo-CT demonstrates adhesive changes in arachnoiditis with the nerve-roots adhering to each other and to the inner surface of the dura mater, and occasionally the spinal cord becomes adherent to the dura in areas of arachnoiditis [79]. These findings can also be expected on high-resolution MRI.

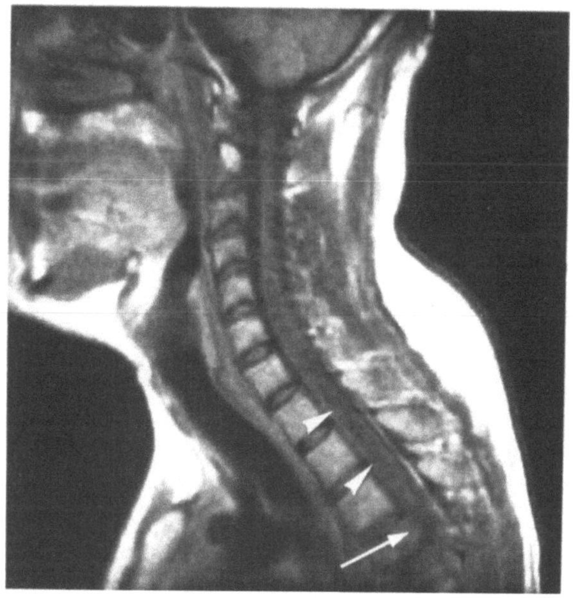

Fig. 72. Posttraumatic syringomyelia *(arrowheads)* above fracture of T4 *(arrow)*. Sagittal T1-weighted MRI

c) Delayed skeletal instability with extradural compression may be another cause of posttraumatic progressive myelopathy [67]. In cervical spinal cord compression, "functional" MRI of the cervical spinal canal can be obtained by recording sagittal images in flexion and extension, showing the mechanism of neural compression [69] (Fig. 24).

d) Posttraumatic microcystic spinal cord degeneration may develop at the site of previous injury and is believed to be a different morphologic entity, manifesting clinically as posttraumatic progressive myelopathy [67]. It has been suggested that it is a consequence of progressive spinal cord ischemia as arachnoiditis encroaches on the blood-supply of the spinal cord. Microcystic myelopathy may mimic syringomyelia not only clinically but also on MRI, especially on T1-weighted images, but unlike the latter it does not respond to shunting. The numerous microcystic fluid-filled cavities honeycombing the cord substance are mistaken for a syrinx on MRI; however, they are assessed correctly by intraoperative ultrasonography. On T2-weighted MR scans, differentiation of microcystic myelopathy from syringomyelia can be attempted: the signal intensity in microcystic degeneration differs from the high intensity found in syringomyelia but is rather similar to that of the surrounding cord substance [97].

Contrary to syringomyelia, microcystic degeneration of the cord tends to be confined to the traumatized level.

e) On rare occasions, gliosis in an atrophic cord can produce progressive posttraumatic myelopathy. The MRI findings are similar to syringomyelia or cyst formation. Proton density images show a high signal intensity [31].

Appendix

A. Diagnostic Procedure

We shall attempt to lay down some guidelines for the rational diagnosis of vertebral fractures, which to a quite substantial extent is a radiologic diagnosis.

I. General Rules

- Always begin with the history and physical examination;
- Technical investigations to be made only if relevant to the treatment;
- Clear concepts of the applicability of a method to the relevant problem. Discussion with clinician;
- Clear statement of problem, to be made intelligible to the radiologist;
- No overdiagnosis. When the examination findings adequately account for the clinical condition of the patient, the diagnosis is completed;
- If possible, cheap rather than costly examinations, and noninvasive rather than invasive.

II. Efficacy of Imaging Methods in Spinal Trauma

1. Plain Film

Radiographic diagnosis in vertebral fractures is extraordinarily competent. Virtually all bony lesions can be detected by approriate projections or tomograms [23]. Of course, such diagnosis of discrete lesions, e. g. of the vertebral arch, calls for great familiarity and reliance on conventional techniques and their radiologic signs. Beyond these, special views and tomograms in acute situations may create problems of time and positioning.

Conventional radiologic diagnosis provides the quickest survey of the spinal column, and the decision whether to employ more elaborate techniques is based on the results. CT and MRI are, so to speak, lenses which permit a more detailed scrutiny of an already recognized pathology.

Advantages:

- rapid localization of fractures,
- high spatial resolution,
- short exposure times and no movement blurring,
- short examination times with restriction to scout views,
- excellent survey of entire structure of spinal column.

Disadvantages:

- problems with superimposition, e. g. blind spot at cervico-thoracic junction,
- discrete lesions of the vertebral arch make great demands on examination technique and assessment,
- tomographs involve relatively higher dosage than CT,
- less soft tissue contrast.

2. Functional Examination

In most cases a spinal injury is left in a spontaneously reduced position which does not correspond exactly to the extent of the original displacement, provided there is no irreducible dislocation or gross destruction.

To assess the load tolerance of the damaged spine in different directions of movement, it must be correspondingly stressed. Plain film radiography is the method of choice. It is capable of demonstrating disko-ligamentous injuries by indirect signs, according to their type, extent and effect on the biomechanics of the spine.

The loading must be done in controlled fashion and should not completely approach the original traumatic deformation. The best control is that of the fully conscious patient himself. Functional diagnosis is not usually urgently indicated, but if for some important reasons it cannot be postponed in patients with clouding or loss of consciousness, it must be done cautiously, gradually and under fluoroscopic supervision. In all other cases it is postponed until the patient is again capable of cooperation. In the meantime, the greatest possible injury based on the diagnostic results so far should be assumed.

The indication for functional views always exists when there is primary or secondary suspicion of a segmental instability from the history, physical examination, course of the condition or imaging techniques.

The contraindication is manifest instability.

Often, functional views in flexion and extension, possibly in lateral flexion also, are adequate. In exceptional cases, rotational views may also be important.

White and Panjabi [115] describe a "stretch test" in which, with the patient supine, gradually increasing axial traction is applied to the spine by pulling on the head up to a load of a third of the body-weight. A lateral radiograph of the affected segment is assessed after each increase in pull. Precise guidelines are given for the performance of the test under medical supervision. The reason for axial stress lies in the relatively great flexibility of the spinal cord in axial movements, whereas the narrowing of the spinal canal associated with lateral displacements naturally tends more to cause complications.

Denis [19] regards as an important sign the widening of the interpeduncular distance in standing views.

Functional assays are also possible using tomographic techniques, or by MRI if there are obscure neurologic symptoms. CT is also advised for functional analysis of the cervico-thoracic junction [25, 26].

The subtle methods of measurement advanced by various authors [3, 10, 86] for the precise analysis of cervical mobility are more suited to the medicolegal field than to the management of acute injury.

Basically, differences between the two sides and (mono-)segmental hyper- and hypomobility and angulation are of particular value in interpreting functional analyses.

3. Computed Tomography

The main advantage of CT for the physician is the absence of superimpositions. The advantage of the greater sharpness of detail has of course to be paid for by the disadvantage of narrowing of the visual field (lens effect).

For the patients, examination in one session after a single positioning in a stable position is very comforting.

Advantages:

- transverse display, especially of the posterior elements, without superimposition,
- easier interpretation of results,
- better soft tissue contrast,
- display of several regions without repositioning.

Disadvantages:

- no overall survey,
- diagnostic difficulties with horizontal fracture-lines (dens fracture),
- time-consuming,
- high costs.

4. Magnetic Resonance Imaging

Though MRI avoids some of the disadvantages of CT, it has fundamental limitations in representing the bones. Attractive features are the great soft tissue contrast, the excellent general overview through optional representational planes and the freedom from ionizing radiation.

Advantages:

- more sensitive than CT in soft tissue injuries,
- the method of choice with obscure neurologic features,

- free choice of representational planes, hence the best general overview,
- no radiation worries,
- MRI myelography without contrast possible.

Disadvantages:

- bony structures difficult to assess,
- hemorrhages in progress difficult to assess,
- difficulties with patient management (intensive care),
- the most expensive and time-consuming examination.

5. Myelography

Myelography is available in several forms: as conventional myelography, CT myelography and MRI myelography. Intrathecal administration of contrast medium is necessary for the first two.

Advantages:

- the best display of the subarachnoid space, including the root pouches.

Disadvantages:

- the most invasive method (except for MRI myelography).

It is mainly indicated for diagnosis of secondary lesions in the subarachnoid space, such as traumatic root avulsion or posttraumatic stenosis of the spinal canal.

III. Sequence of Examinations

On the basis of our experience, we proceed as follows. As already mentioned, a staged diagnostic program should be observed. At each stage a check should be made to see whether the existing findings adequately account for the clinical features. If not, the clinical and therapeutic implications should be considered before further examinations.

If they do, the diagnostic procedure should be terminated, unless more detailed information is required for operative management.

Three categories of patients may be distinguished according to the urgency of treatment:

a) those that can be managed electively, with risks neither to life nor neurologic status,
b) those requiring urgent management but with stable vital functions
c) those at risk of life.

"Neurologic risk" implies that serious neurologic damage is to be feared but has not yet developed, or that there exists a potentially reversible neurologic lesion.

The more urgent the situation, the earlier should CT be employed, in exceptional cases even without radiographic views. CT is particularly useful where several regions of the body must be examined at the same time.

1. Diagnostic Imaging in Elective Treatment

- plain films, possibly with special projections and tomographs,
- functional diagnosis,
- CT where the bony and/or neurologic situation is obscure,
- secondary MRI if the findings in CT do not account for the neurologic picture,
- myelography in the event of persistent problems concerning the subarachnoid space and nerve-roots (e. g. in plexus avulsion).

2. Diagnostic Imaging in Urgent Treatment

- plain views,
- cranial CT in unconscious patients,
- CT of the spine in obscure bony and/or neurologic conditions,
- MRI in obscure neurologic conditions.

3. Diagnostic Imaging in Life-threatening Lesions

- plain film of the thorax and abdominal ultrasonography accompanying intensive care to stabilize vital functions,
- CT orientation, possibly of several regions (head, thorax, abdomen), display of subsidiary areas by scout view/topogram,
- after clinical stabilization, as under one of the two categories above.

References

1. Allen BL, Ferguson RL, Lehmann TR, O'Brian RP (1982) A mechanistic classification of closed indirect fractures and dislocations of the lower cervical spine. Spine 7: 1-27
2. Anderson LD, D'Alonzo RT (1974) Fracture of the odontoid process of the axis. J Bone J Surg 56-A: 1663-1674
3. Arlen A (1979) Biometrische Röntgen-Funktionsdiagnostik der Halswirbelsäule. Man Med 5, Fischer, Heidelberg
4. Beers GJ, Raque GH, Wagner GG, Shields CB, Nichols GR, Johnson JR, Meyer JE (1988) MR imaging in acute cervical spine trauma. JCAT 12,5: 755-761
5. Bohlman HH, Ducker TB, Lucas JT (1982) Spine and spinal cord injuries. In: Rothman RH, Simeone FA (eds) The spine. W. B. Saunders Company, Philadelphia
6. Brachlow M (1984) Zur Computertomographie der Wirbelsaulenverletzungen. Symposium "Spinale Computertomographie", 45-49
7. Buchanan LE, Nawoczenski DA (1987) Spinal cord injury. Concepts and management approaches. Williams & Wilkins, Baltimore
8. Buchholz RW (1981) Unstable hangman's fractures. Clin Orthop 154: 119-124
9. Buchholz RW, Gill K (1986) Classification of injuries to the thoraco-lumbar spine. Orthop Clin North Am 17: 67-73
10. Buetti-Bauml C (1954) Funktionelle Diagnostik der Halswirbelsäule. Thieme, Stuttgart
11. Burguet JL, Sick H, Dirheimer Y, Wackenheim A (1985) CT of the main ligaments of the cervico-occipital hinge. Neuroradiology 27: 112-118
12. Calenoff L, Chessare JW, Rogers LF, Toerge J, Rosen JS (1978) Multiple level spinal injuries: importance of early recognition. Amer J Roentgenol 130: 665-669
13. Chance GQ (1948) Note on a type of flexion fracture of the spine. Br J Radiol 2: 452-453
14. Clark CR, White AA (1985) Fractures of the dens. A multicenter study. J Bone Joint Surg 67-A: 1340-1348
15. Clyburn TA, Lionberger DR, Tullos HS (1982) Bilateral fracture of the transverse process of the atlas. J Bone Joint Surg 64-A: 948
16. Cooper PR, Cohen W (1984) Evaluation of cervical spinal cord injuries with metrizamide myelography-CT scanning. J Neurosurg 61: 281-289
17. Crone-Münzenbrock W, Jend HH, Heller M, Schöttle H (1984) Spinal fractures: results and experience with computer tomography. Arch Orthop Trauma Surg 103: 36-41
18. Daßbach A, Hamacher E, Neubert H (1983) Arbeits- und Wegeunfälle in der medizinischen Rehabilitation. Statistik über verletzte Körperteile, Verletzungsarten und Verletzungsfolgen. Hauptverband der gewerblichen Berufsgenossenschaften eV (Hrsg), Bonn
19. Denis F (1983) The three column spine and its significance in the classification of acute thoracolumbar spinal injuries. Spine 8: 817-831
20. Denis F (1984) Spinal instability as defined by the three-column spine concept in acute spinal trauma. Clin Orthop 189: 65-76
21. Denis F, Armstrong GW, Searls K, Matta L (1984) Acute thoracolumbar burst fractures in the absence of neurologic deficit. A comparison between operative and nonoperative treatment. Clin Orthop 189: 142-149
22. Dorr LD, Harvey JP, Nickel VL (1982) Clinical review of the early stability of spine injuries. Spine 7: 545-550
23. Dosch JC (1985) Trauma. Conventional radiological study in spine injury. Springer, Berlin, Heidelberg, New York, Tokyo
24. Ducker TB, Lucas JT, Wallace CA (1983) Recovery from spinal cord injury. In: Weiss MH (ed) Clinical neurosurgery, vol 30. William & Wilkins, Baltimore
25. Dvorak J, Hayek J (1986) Diagnostik der Instabilität der oberen Halswirbelsäule mittels funktioneller Computertomographie. Fortschr Rontgenstr 145: 582-585
26. Dvorak J, Penning L, Hayek J, Panjabi MM, Grob D, Zehnder R (1988) Functional diagnostics of the cervical spine using computer tomography. Neuroradiology 30: 132-137
27. Effendi B, Roy D, Cornish B, Dussault RG, Laurin CA (1981) Fractures of the ring of the axis. J Bone Joint Surg 63-B: 319-327
28. Farfan HF (1973) Mechanical disorders of the low back. Lea & Fibiger, Philadelphia
29. Farfan HF, Gracovetzky S (1984) The nature of instability. Spine 9: 714-719
30. Ferguson RL, Allen BL (1984) A mechanistic classification of thoracolumbar spine fractures. Clin Orthop 189: 77-88
31. Fox JL, Wener L, Drennan DC, Manz HJ, Won DJ, Al-Mefty O (1988) Central spinal cord injury: magnetic resonance imaging confirmation and operative considerations. Neurosurgery 22: 340-347
32. Frankel HL, Hancock DO, Hyslop G (1969) The value of postural reduction in initial management of closed injuries of the spine with paraplegia and tetraplegia. Paraplegia 7: 179-192
33. Gebarski SS, Maynard FW, Gabrielsen TO, Knake JE, Latack JT, Hoff JT (1985) Posttraumatic progressive myelopathy. Radiology 157: 379-385
34. Gehweiler JA, Duff DE, Martinez S, Miller MD, Clark WM (1976) Fractures of the atlas vertebra. Skeletal Radiol 1: 97-102

35. Gracovetzky S, Farfan HF, Lamy C (1981) The mechanism of the lumbar spine. Spine 6: 249-262
36. Gracovetzky S, Farfan HF, Helleur C (1985) The abdominal mechanism. Spine 10: 317-324
37. Gracovetzky S, Farfan H (1986) The optimum spine. Spine 11: 543-573
38. Green BA, Magana IA (1987) Spinal cord trauma: clinical aspects. In: Davidoff RA (ed) Handbook of the spinal cord. Marcel Decker, New York
39. Hackney DB, Asato R, Joseph PM, Carvlin MJ, McGrath JT, Grossman RI, Kassab EA, DeSimone D (1986) Hemorrhage and edema in acute spinal cord compression: demonstration by MR imaging. Radiology 161: 387-390
40. Hardy AG, Rossier AB (1975) Spinal cord injuries. Thieme, Stuttgart
41. Harris JH, Burge JT, Ray RD, Nichols-Hostetter S, Lester RG (1984) Low (type III) odontoid fracture: a new radiographic sign. Radiology 153: 353-356
42. Haughton VM, Syvertsen A, Williams AL (1980) Soft-tissue anatomy within the spinal canal as seen on computed tomography. Radiology 134: 649-655
43. Haughton VM, Williams AL (1982) Computed tomography of the spine. CV Mosby Co, St Louis
44. Haughton VM, Daniels DL, Czervionke LF, Williams AL (1988) Cervical spine. In: Stark DD, Bradley WG (eds) Magnetic resonance imaging. CV Mosby Co, St Louis
45. Herkowitz HN, Rothmann RH (1984) Subacute instability of the cervical spine. Spine 9: 348-357
46. Holdsworth F (1970) Fractures, dislocations, and fracture-dislocations of the spine. J Bone Joint Surg 52-A: 1534-1551
47. Imhof H, Hajek P, Kumpan W, Schratter M, Wagner M (1986) CT in der Akutdiagnostik von Wirbelsaulentraumen. Radiologe 26: 242-247
48. Jaeger R, Whitely WH (1953) Avulsion of the brachial plexus. JAMA 153: 644-649
49. Jellinger K (1976) Neuropathology of cord injuries. In: Vinken PJ, Bruyn GW (eds) Handbook of clinical neurology. Vol 25. North-Holland Publ, Amsterdam
50. Jodoin A, Dupuis P, Fraser M, Beaumont P (1985) Unstable fractures of the thoracolumbar spine: a 10-year experience at Sacré-Coeur Hospital. J Traum 25: 197-202
51. Kadoya S, Nakamura T, Kobayashi S, Yamamoto I (1987) Magnetic resonance of acute spinal cord injury. Neuroradiology 29: 252-255
52. Kahle W, Leonhard H, Platzer W (1979) Taschenatlas der Anatomie. Thieme, Stuttgart
53. Kalfas I, Wilberger J, Goldberg A, Prostko ER (1988) Magnetic resonance imaging in acute spinal cord trauma. Neurosurgery 23: 295-299
54. Kim KS, Rogers LF, Regenbogen V (1986) Pitfalls in plain film diagnosis of cervical spine injuries: false positive interpretation. Surg Neurol 25: 381-392
55. Kirkaldy-Willis WH, Farfan HF (1982) Instability of the lumbar spine. Clin Orthop 165: 110-123
56. Kocks W, Kalff R, Roosen K, Grote W (1986) Spina Bifida Anterior Atlantis - Fehlinterpretation einer angeborenen Mißbildung als Dens-Fraktur. Unfallchirurg 89: 142-144
57. Kohler A, Zimmer EA (1982) Grenzen des Normalen und Anfänge des Pathologischen im Röntgenbild des Skeletts. Thieme, Stuttgart
58. Krämer J (1986) Bandscheibenbedingte Erkrankungen. Thieme, Stuttgart
59. Kulkarni MV, McArdle CB, Kopanicky D, Miner M, Cotler HB, Lee KF, Harris JH (1987) Acute spinal cord injury: MR imaging at 1.5 T. Radiology 164: 837-843
60. Kulkarni MV, Bondurant FJ, Rose SL, Narayana PA (1988) 1.5 Tesla magnetic resonance imaging of acute spinal trauma. RadioGraphics 8: 1059-1082
61. Kuner EH (1986) Verletzungen im Brust-Lendenwirbelsäulen-Bereich. Klassifikation und klinisch-neurologische Diagnostik. In: Godecke AG (Hrsg): 18. Freiburger Chirurgengesprach: 98-110
62. Lange S, Grumme T, Kluge W, Ringel K, Meese W (1988) Zerebrale und spinale Computertomographie. Schering AG, Berlin
63. Levitan LH, Wiens CW (1983) Chronic lumbar extradural hematoma: CT findings. Radiology 148: 707-708
64. Leyendecker K, Schırmer M (1985) Traumatische Rückenmarkschädigungen. In: Schirmer M (ed) Querschnittslahmungen. Springer, Berlin, Heidelberg, New York, Tokyo
65. Lindahl O (1976) Mechanical properties of dried defattied spongy bone Acta Orthop Scand 47: 11
66. Louis R (1985) Die Chirurgie der Wirbelsäule. Springer, Berlin, Heidelberg, New York, Tokyo
67. Macdonald RL, Findlay MJ, Tator CH (1988) Microcystic spinal cord degeneratıon causing posttraumatic myelopathy. J Neurosurg 68: 466-471
68. McAfee PC, Yuan HA, Frederickson BE, Lubicky JP (1983) The value of computed tomography in thoracolumbar fractures. An analysis of one hundred consecutive cases and a new classification. J Bone Joint Surg 65-A: 461-473
69. McAfee PC, Bohlman HH, Han JS, Salvagno RT (1986) Comparison of nuclear magnetic resonance imaging and computed tomography ın the diagnosis of upper cervical spinal cord compression. Spıne 11: 295-304
70. McArdle CB, Crofford MJ, Mirfakhraee M, Amparo EG, Calhoun JS (1986) Surface coil MR of spinal trauma: preliminary experience. AJNR 7: 885-893
71. Magerl F (1985) Der Wirbel-Fixateur externe. In: Weber BG, Magerl F (Hrsg) Fixateur externe. Springer, Heidelberg, Berlin, New York, Tokyo
72. Mark AS, Scott WA (1988) MRI of the cervical spine and cord. MRI decisions 2: 23-32
73. Markolf KL, Morris JM (1974) The structural components of the intervertebral disc. J Bone Joint Surg 56-A: 675-687
74. Meuli H (1980) Röntgenuntersuchung der verletzten Wirbelsäule. Orthopäde 9: 7-15
75. Mirvis SE, Geisler FH, Jelinek JJ, Joslyn JN, Gellad F (1988) Acute cervical spine trauma: evaluation with 1.5 T MR imaging. Radiology 166: 807-816
76. Modic MT, Hardy RW, Weınstein MA, Duchesneau PM, Paushter DM, Boumfrey F (1984) Nuclear magnetic resonance imagıng of the spine: clinical potential and limitation. Neurosurgery 15: 583-592
77. Morris RE, Hasso AN, Thompson JR, Hinshaw DB, Vu LH (1984) Traumatic dural tears: CT diagnosis using metrizamide. Radiology 152: 443-446
78. Nachemson A, Morris JM (1964) In vivo measurements of intradiskal pressure. J Bone Joint Surg 46: 1077-1092
79. Newton TH, Potts DG (1983) Computed tomography of the spine and spinal cord. Clavadel Press, San Anselmo
80. Norman D (1987) The spine. In: Brant-Zawadzki M,

Norman D (eds) Magnetic resonance imaging of the central nervous system. Raven press, New York
81. Noyes FR, DeLucas JL, Torvik PJ (1974) Biomechanics of anterior cruciate ligament failure: an analysis of strain-rate sensitivity and mechanisms of failure in primates. J Bone Joint Surg 56A: 236-253
82. Oliveira E, Rhoton AL, Peace D (1985) Microsurgical anatomy of the foramen magnum. Surg Neurol 24: 293-352
83. Pan G, Kulkarni M, MacDougall DJ, Miner ME (1988) Traumatic epidural hematoma of the cervical spine: Diagnosis with magnetic resonance imaging. J Neurosurg 68: 798-801
84. Panjabi MM, Brand RA, White (III) AA (1976) Mechanical properties of the human thoracic spine. J Bone Joint Surg 60-A: 481-488
85. Panjabi MM, Krag MH, Chung TQ (1984) Effects of disc injury on mechanical behaviour of the human spine. Spine 9: 707-713
86. Penning L (1978) Normal movements of the cervical spine. AJR 130: 317-326
87. Penning L (1981) Prevertebral hematoma in cervical spine injury: incidence and etiologic significance. AJR 136: 553-561
88. Pepin JW, Hawkins RJ (1981) Traumatic spondylolisthesis of the axis: hangman's fracture. Clin Orthop 157: 133-138
89. Plaue R (1973) Die Mechanik des Wirbelkompressionsbruchs. Zentralbl Chir 98: 761-770
90. Pojunas K, Williams AL, Daniels DL, Haughton VM (1984) Syringomyelia and hydromyelia: magnetic resonance evaluation. Radiology 153: 679-683
91. Pope MH, Panjabi MM (1985) Biomechanical definitions of spinal instability. Spine 10: 255-256
92 Post JD, Seminer DS, Quencer TM (1982) CT diagnosis of spinal epidural hematoma. AJNR 3: 190-192
93. Post JD (1984) Computed tomography of the spine. Williams & Wilkins, Baltimore
94. Prestar FJ, Putz R (1982) Das Ligamentum longitudinale posterius. Morphologie und Funktion. Morphol Med 2: 181-189
95. Putz R (1983) Zur Morphologie und Dynamik der Wirbelsäule. Radiologe 23: 145-150
96. Quencer RM, Green BA, Eismont FJ (1983) Posttraumatic spinal cord cysts: clinical features and characterization with metrizamide computed tomography. Radiology 146: 415-423
97. Quencer RM, Sheldon JJ, Post JD, Diaz RD, Montalvo BM, Green BA, Eismont FJ (1986) MRI of the chronically injured cervical spinal cord. AJR 147: 125-132
98. Raynor RB, Koplik B (1985) Cervical cord trauma. The relationships between clinical syndromes and force injury. Spine 10: 193-197
99. Regenbogen VS, Rogers LF, Atlas SW, Kim KS (1986) Cervical spinal cord injuries in patients with cervical spondylosis. AJR 146: 277-284
100. Roy-Camille R, Saillant C, Berteaux D, Marie-Anne S (1979) Early management of spinal injuries. In: McKibbin B (ed) Recent advances in orthopedics. Churchill Livingstone, Edinburgh, London
101. Ruge D, Wiltse LL (1977) Spinal disorders. Lea & Febiger, Philadelphia
102. Saternus KS, Paul E (1986) Bruchformen des Dens axis bei ventralflektierender Krafteinleitung. Akt Traumatol 16: 28-33
103. Saternus KS, Thrun C (1987) Zur Traumatologie der Ligamenta alaria. Akt Traumatol 17: 214-218
104. Schild H, Schweden F, Weigand H (1982) Horizontalfraktur des ventralen Atlasbogens. Fortschr Röntgenstr 136: 485-486
105. Schirmer M (1985) Der spinale Notfall. Perimed Fachbuch-Verlagsgesellschaft, Erlangen
106. Schmorl G, Junghanns H (1968) Die gesunde und die kranke Wirbelsäule in Röntgenbild und Klinik. Thieme, Stuttgart
107. Schützhoff G (1988) Behandlungskonzept und Resultate bei Frakturen der unteren Brust- und Lendenwirbelsäule. Inaugural-Dissertation, Albert-Ludwigs-Universität, Freiburg
108. Seibert CE, Dreisbach JN, Swanson WB, Edgar RE, Williams P, Hahn H (1981) Progressive posttraumatic cystic myelopathy: neuroradiologic evaluation. AJR 136: 1161-1165
109. Signoret F, Feron JM, Bonfait H, Patel A (1986) Fractured odontoid with fractured superior articular process of the axis. J Bone Joint Surg 68-B: 182-184
110. Smith WS, Kaufer H (1969) Patterns and mechanisms of lumbar injuries associated with lap seat belts. J Bone Joint Surg 51-A: 239-254
111. Tarr RW, Drolshagen LF, Kerner TC, Allen JH, Partain CL, James EA (1987) MR imaging of recent spinal trauma. JCAT 11: 412-417
112. Tkaczuk H (1968) Tensile properties of human lumbar longitudinal ligaments. Acta Orthop Scand 115 (Suppl)
113. Trafton PG, Boyd CA (1984) Computed tomography of thoracic and lumbar spine injuries. J Trauma 24: 506-515
114. Virgin W (1951) Experimental investigations into the physical properties of the intervertebral disc. J Bone Joint Surg 33-B: 607-611
115. White AA, Panjabi MM (1978) Clinical biomechanics of the spine. Lippincott, Philadelphia
116. Wimmer B, Friedburg H, Hennig J, Kauffmann GW (1986) Möglichkeiten der diagnostischen Bildgebung durch Kernspintomographie. Veränderungen an Wirbeln, Bandern und Bandscheiben im Vergleich mit der Computertomographie. Radiologe 26: 137-143
117. Wittenberg HR, Beyer HK, Bötel U (1987) Magnetische Resonanztomographie der Halswirbelsäule bei vollständiger Querschnittslähmung. Fortschr Röntgenstr 147: 352-354
118. Zilkha A, Irwin GA, Fagelmann D (1983) Computed tomography of acute spinal epidural hematoma. AJNR 4: 1073-1076

Subject Index

Page numbers referring to figures are given in *italics*